Schema Therapy for Young Adults

The Complete Guide to Healing the Emotional Patterns That Control Your Life

I0145223

May Ivette Ray

Table of Contents

Chapter 1: Your Patterns Are Forming Right Now - Why Young Adulthood Matters

The years between eighteen and thirty represent something extraordinary in human development. During this period, your brain undergoes its final major renovation project—one that shapes who you become for the rest of your life. The patterns you establish now, the ways you learn to cope with stress, relate to others, and view yourself, are literally being wired into your neural architecture. This isn't just psychological theory; it's biological fact.

Your Brain Is Still Under Construction (And That's Amazing)

Most people assume brain development stops somewhere around high school graduation. The reality is far more interesting. Your prefrontal cortex—the brain's CEO responsible for decision-making, impulse control, and long-term planning—continues developing well into your late twenties[1]. This extended construction period means you're operating with a brain that's simultaneously more flexible and more vulnerable than it will ever be again.

Consider Maya, a twenty-four-year-old marketing coordinator who found herself saying yes to every request at work, staying late to help colleagues, and apologizing constantly for things that weren't her fault. She'd been the family peacekeeper since age eight, when her parents' marriage hit rocky ground. Back then, being helpful meant less fighting at home. Now, sixteen years later, her brain had turned this survival strategy into automatic programming.

Every time someone seemed disappointed or frustrated, Maya's neural pathways fired the same message: "Fix it. Make them happy. Keep the peace."

This automatic response wasn't just habit—it was literally carved into her brain's wiring through years of repetition during critical developmental periods. The good news? At twenty-four, Maya's brain still possessed enough plasticity to create new pathways, new patterns, new ways of being in the world.

The Schema Formation Sweet Spot

Schemas—those deep-seated patterns of thinking, feeling, and behaving—typically form during childhood as ways to cope with our environment[2]. But here's what most people don't realize: young adulthood represents a unique window where these schemas become more entrenched while simultaneously remaining malleable enough to change. You're in the schema formation sweet spot.

Think of schemas like well-worn paths through a forest. During childhood, you create these paths based on what helps you survive and get your needs met. By young adulthood, these paths have become highways—efficient, automatic routes your brain takes without conscious thought. But unlike actual highways, neural pathways can still be rerouted during this developmental window.

Jake's story illustrates this perfectly. At twenty-seven, he'd ended three potentially serious relationships at exactly the six-month mark. Each time, as soon as his partner started talking about future plans or leaving belongings at his apartment, Jake felt an overwhelming urge to run. His abandonment schema, formed when his father left without warning when Jake was nine, had created a protective pattern: leave before you can be left.

What Jake didn't realize was that his brain was operating on outdated software. The abandonment he feared had already happened, nearly two decades ago. But his neural pathways didn't know that. They were still running the same protective program, like a computer virus that keeps executing even when the original threat is long gone.

Breaking Free from Autopilot Mode

Young adults often feel like they're sleepwalking through life, making decisions that don't quite feel like their own. This autopilot mode isn't laziness or lack of ambition—it's your schemas running the show. The brain loves efficiency, and nothing is more efficient than following pre-programmed patterns.

Aisha discovered this at twenty-five when she realized her entire life looked perfect on Instagram but felt empty in reality. She had 10,000 followers who loved her curated apartment tours, outfit posts, and motivational quotes. But behind the camera, Aisha was drowning in credit card debt, struggling with intense loneliness, and feeling like a fraud. Her "defectiveness" schema—the deep belief that she was fundamentally flawed—drove her to create an online persona that was everything she believed she wasn't: confident, successful, worthy of admiration.

The energy required to maintain this false self was exhausting. Every post required hours of preparation, editing, and anxiety about reception. The dopamine hits from likes and comments provided temporary relief from her core belief of being defective, but like any quick fix, it never lasted. The schema always returned, demanding more proof, more perfection, more external validation.

Breaking free from autopilot requires first recognizing that you're on it. Most young adults don't realize how much of their behavior is schema-driven until they start paying attention. That moment of recognition—"Wait, I'm doing it again"—is the beginning of change.

Your Quarter-Life Crisis Is Actually Your Brain Upgrading

The term "quarter-life crisis" gets thrown around like it's something to be fixed or avoided. In reality, this period of confusion, questioning, and discomfort is your brain's way of upgrading its operating system[3]. The uncertainty you feel isn't a bug—it's a feature.

During this developmental phase, your brain is simultaneously consolidating what it's learned while remaining open to new information and experiences[4]. This creates a unique psychological state where you're aware enough to question your patterns but still flexible enough to change them. The discomfort comes from existing in this in-between space—no longer who you were, not yet who you're becoming.

David exemplified this perfectly. At twenty-six, he found himself in his fourth job in three years, each change prompted by a vague sense that something wasn't right. His friends called him flaky. His parents worried about his lack of direction. David himself felt like a failure, especially compared to peers who seemed to have their lives figured out.

What David was actually experiencing was his brain's attempt to reconcile his authentic self with the schemas he'd developed. His "unrelenting standards" schema, formed in a household where anything less than perfection meant criticism, was clashing with his emerging adult identity. Each job change represented his psyche's attempt to find a fit between who he was expected to be and who he actually was.

The Schema Healing Advantage: Why Now Is Your Time

The convergence of continued brain plasticity, schema consolidation, and adult self-awareness creates an unprecedented opportunity for change during young adulthood[5]. You have advantages that neither children nor older adults possess: enough life experience to recognize patterns, sufficient brain flexibility to change them, and the motivation that comes from wanting to build your own life.

Research in neuroplasticity shows that while the brain remains changeable throughout life, the effort required to create new neural pathways increases with age[6]. In your twenties, your brain is still naturally prone to forming new connections. It's like the difference between learning a language at twenty-five versus fifty-five—both are possible, but one requires significantly less effort.

Emma discovered this advantage when she began working with her patterns at twenty-three. Her "emotional inhibition" schema made her appear cold and distant, even though she desperately wanted close friendships. Growing up in a family where emotions were seen as weakness, Emma had learned to lock her feelings away so thoroughly that she couldn't access them even when she wanted to.

The work wasn't easy, but Emma's young adult brain was primed for it. Within six months of conscious practice—

sharing one genuine feeling per day, allowing herself to cry during movies, telling friends when they hurt her feelings—Emma noticed significant changes. Her neural pathways, still flexible from ongoing development, adapted more quickly than they would have a decade later.

This isn't to say change becomes impossible after thirty. But right now, in this developmental sweet spot, you have neurological advantages that make schema healing more accessible and potentially more profound. Your brain is literally designed to revolutionize itself during this period.

Taking Action: Your Schema Healing Toolkit

Understanding the theory is important, but change happens through action. The following exercises are designed to work with, not against, your developing brain:

The Schema Journal: Starting today, keep a simple record of moments when you feel triggered, reactive, or like you're operating on autopilot. Note the situation, your emotional response, and any patterns you recognize. This isn't about judgment—it's about developing schema awareness.

Pattern Detective Practice: For one week, approach your life like an anthropologist studying human behavior. When you react strongly to something, ask yourself: "How old do I feel right now?" Often, schema-driven responses make us feel much younger than our actual age. That's your clue that you're dealing with an old pattern, not a current reality.

Brain Timeline Mapping: Create a visual timeline of your life, marking significant events and the coping strategies you developed in response. Look for connections between past adaptations and current behaviors. Remember, every schema served a purpose once—the question is whether it's still serving you now.

Schema Trigger Tracking: Identify three situations that consistently trigger strong reactions. These might be criticism at work, romantic partners pulling away, or social media comparison. These triggers are pointing directly to your schemas. Once you know what triggers you, you can prepare different responses.

Neuroplasticity Promise Letter: Write a letter to yourself acknowledging that change is possible. Include specific patterns you want to address and remind yourself that your brain is literally designed to create new pathways right now. Read this letter whenever schema work feels too hard.

The journey of schema healing in young adulthood isn't about fixing something broken—it's about updating your internal software to match who you're becoming. Your brain is ready for this work. The patterns that protected you in childhood don't have to define your adulthood. This developmental window won't stay open forever, but right now, it's wide open. The question isn't whether change is possible; it's whether you're ready to begin.

Key Takeaways

- Your brain continues developing through your late twenties, creating a unique window for pattern change that combines neural flexibility with adult awareness

- Schemas formed in childhood become more entrenched during young adulthood but remain malleable enough to modify with conscious effort

- The "quarter-life crisis" is actually your brain upgrading its operating system—the discomfort signals growth, not failure

- Young adults have neurological advantages for schema healing that decrease with age, making this the optimal time for deep pattern work

- Recognizing schema-driven behaviors is the first step toward change; awareness creates choice where there was once only automatic reaction

Chapter 2: The Approval Addiction - Social Media and Validation Schemas

Every notification carries a promise. The gentle buzz of your phone suggests that somewhere, someone has noticed you, approved of you, validated your existence. For young adults who grew up alongside social media, this constant stream of potential approval has created an entirely new arena for ancient human needs to play out. The approval schemas that once operated in family systems and small communities now perform on a global digital stage.

Welcome to the Validation Economy

Social media platforms haven't just changed how we communicate—they've fundamentally altered how we measure our worth[7]. In this new economy, likes are currency, followers are status, and engagement rates determine value. For young adults whose brains are still developing their sense of identity, this external measurement system can hijack the natural process of self-discovery.

The platforms themselves are engineered to exploit our neurological wiring. Every like triggers a small hit of dopamine, the same neurotransmitter involved in addiction[8]. The variable ratio reinforcement—never knowing when the next approval hit will come—keeps us scrolling, posting, checking. It's not weakness that keeps you returning to these apps; it's sophisticated behavioral design meeting vulnerable neural pathways.

Chloe learned this the hard way. A twenty-three-year-old graphic designer, she would post her artwork on Instagram with trembling fingers, then refresh obsessively for the first hour. If a post didn't hit fifty likes within that window, she'd delete it. The shame felt physical—a tightness in her chest, heat flooding her face. What Chloe didn't realize was that each deleted post reinforced her approval-seeking schema, teaching her brain that her worth was determined by digital metrics.

The worst part? The posts that got the most likes were rarely her favorites. The algorithm rewarded conformity, predictability, hashtag optimization—not authenticity or artistic risk. Chloe found herself creating two portfolios: one for Instagram approval, another of work she actually cared about but never shared.

Your Childhood Approval Needs Meet Instagram

Every adult carries within them the child who first learned what it took to be loved. For some, love meant achievement. For others, it meant being helpful, or funny, or invisible. These early lessons create templates—schemas—that determine how we seek approval throughout life[9]. Social media provides a 24/7 laboratory for these patterns to express themselves.

Marcus discovered his LinkedIn had become a digital recreation of his childhood dinner table. Growing up as the eldest son of immigrant parents, he'd learned that worth came through accomplishment. Report cards were scrutinized, awards were expected, and anything less than excellence meant disappointment. Now at twenty-six, Marcus found himself crafting LinkedIn posts about every minor work achievement, checking obsessively for reactions and comments from professional connections he'd never met.

The pattern was exhausting but familiar. Just as he'd once brought home grades for parental approval, he now offered up professional updates for digital validation. The likes felt momentarily satisfying, like his father's rare nod of approval. But also like that childhood approval, it was never enough. There was always another achievement to share, another metric to hit, another way to prove his worth.

What made it worse was watching peers post about their successes. Each announcement of a promotion or new job triggered the same competitive anxiety he'd felt with his siblings. The platform turned professional life into a performance, complete with an audience keeping score.

The Comparison Trap and Your Developing Identity

Young adulthood is naturally a time of identity exploration and social comparison. You're figuring out who you are partly by observing who others are[10]. Social media amplifies this natural process into something potentially toxic, offering unlimited opportunities for upward comparison with curated versions of others' lives.

The comparison trap operates on a fundamental unfairness: you're comparing your inner experience with others' external presentation. You know your own struggles, doubts, and failures intimately. You see only what others choose to show. This asymmetry of information creates a perception gap that feeds directly into schemas of defectiveness, failure, or inadequacy.

Zara, at twenty-five, had turned Instagram story-watching into a form of digital self-harm. She'd wake up and immediately check who had viewed her stories from the night before, analyzing who had skipped through quickly and who had watched to the end. Then she'd move on to watching others' stories, each one a small wound: the college friend traveling through Bali, the coworker's perfect apartment, the high school acquaintance's engagement announcement.

By the time Zara got out of bed, she'd already spent thirty minutes reinforcing her "defectiveness/shame" schema. Everyone else seemed to have figured out adult life while she was still struggling with basics. What Zara couldn't see was that many of those people were doing their own comparison scroll, feeling inadequate about different things. The platform created a circular firing squad of insecurity.

Breaking the Scroll-Validate-Crash Cycle

The pattern is predictable: post something, feel anxious, check repeatedly for validation, feel temporarily satisfied or deeply disappointed, crash into shame or emptiness, scroll through others' content for distraction, feel worse, post something to feel better, repeat. This cycle can consume hours daily and years of young adult life.

Breaking free requires understanding both the neurological and psychological mechanisms at play. Your brain has been trained to expect and crave these dopamine hits[11]. Your schemas have found a perfect playground for their patterns. But neither of these facts makes you powerless.

The first step is pattern interruption. When Marcus realized he was checking LinkedIn every ten minutes during work, he implemented a simple intervention: before each check, he had to write down what he hoped to find. "Seven people liked my post about the quarterly report." "My manager commented on my certification announcement." Seeing these hopes written out helped him recognize the futility—no amount of professional validation would fill the childhood wound of conditional love.

Chloe took a different approach. She started posting her real work—the weird, experimental pieces that made her nervous—with comments disabled. This removed the immediate feedback loop while still allowing her to share. Over time, she noticed something interesting: without the metric of likes, she had to develop her own sense of what was good. Her artistic voice, muffled by the need for approval, began to emerge.

Building Your Internal Validation System

The opposite of external validation isn't no validation—it's internal validation. This doesn't mean becoming a narcissist who needs no one else's input. It means developing a stable sense of self-worth that external feedback can inform but not define[12].

Internal validation is a skill that requires practice, especially for those with strong approval-seeking schemas. It involves learning to recognize and appreciate your own efforts, progress, and inherent worth outside of any performance metrics. For young adults who've grown up in the validation economy, this can feel like learning to breathe in a new atmosphere.

Zara began with a simple practice: each night before bed, she wrote down three things she'd done that day that aligned with her values, regardless of whether anyone noticed. "I helped my anxious coworker with her presentation." "I chose to cook dinner instead of ordering out." "I called my grandmother." These weren't Instagram-worthy moments, but they were expressions of who Zara wanted to be.

The practice felt forced at first, her schema insisting these small acts didn't count without external witness. But gradually, Zara developed an internal witness—a part of herself that could recognize and validate her own experiences. This didn't eliminate her desire for connection and recognition, but it provided a stable foundation that social media metrics couldn't shake.

Practical Strategies for Schema-Aware Social Media Use

Living in the digital age doesn't require digital abstinence. The goal isn't to eliminate social media but to use it in ways that support rather than sabotage your psychological development. Here are evidence-based strategies for maintaining your mental health while staying connected:

The Three-Day Validation Audit: Track every instance of seeking or receiving digital validation for three days. Include posting, checking for responses, viewing others' content, and the emotions involved. This creates a data-based picture of your patterns without judgment.

Implement the Phone Check Protocol: Designate specific times for social media checks rather than constant monitoring. Start with three scheduled checks daily, then adjust based on what feels sustainable. The goal is intentional rather than compulsive use.

Create Validation-Free Zones: Establish physical spaces and time periods where validation-seeking is off-limits. This might be your bedroom, the first hour after waking, or during meals. These zones allow your nervous system to remember what it feels like to exist without external measurement.

Design Your Feed Mindfully: Unfollow or mute accounts that consistently trigger comparison or inadequacy. Follow accounts that inspire genuine growth rather than schema activation. Your feed should feel like a supportive friend, not a critical judge.

Practice Real-World Validation: For every digital validation sought, balance it with a real-world connection. Text a friend directly instead of posting for many. Share accomplishments with someone who matters rather than broadcasting to strangers. This helps maintain the human element in your need for connection.

The rise of social media has created unprecedented challenges for young adult development. Never before have so many people had their worth measured so publicly and constantly. But within this challenge lies opportunity. By becoming conscious of how digital platforms interact with your schemas, you can use these tools rather than being used by them. Your worth existed before your first post and will persist after your last. The validation you seek through screens is a poor substitute for the acceptance you can learn to give yourself.

Key Takeaways

- Social media platforms are designed to exploit approval-seeking behaviors through sophisticated behavioral psychology, creating addictive cycles that reinforce validation schemas

- Childhood patterns of seeking love and approval find new expression through digital platforms, often recreating family dynamics in online spaces

- The comparison trap of social media creates unfair measurements by comparing your internal reality with others' curated external presentations

- Breaking validation addiction requires conscious pattern interruption and the development of internal validation skills that exist independent of metrics

- Strategic social media use involves creating boundaries, mindful consumption, and balancing digital interaction with real-world connection

Chapter 3: Quarter-Life Crisis Decoded - Identity and Direction Confusion

The email arrives on a Tuesday morning. Your college roommate just got promoted to senior manager at a company you've never heard of but sounds impressive. You're sitting at a desk that feels temporary, in a job that feels like a placeholder, living a life that feels like a rough draft. The voice in your head gets louder: "Everyone else has it figured out. What's wrong with me?"

This is the quarter-life crisis in action—that peculiar cocktail of anxiety, confusion, and existential dread that hits somewhere between your first real job and your thirtieth birthday[13]. But what if this crisis isn't a problem to be solved but a developmental process to be understood?

Your Crisis Is Actually a Cocoon

The quarter-life crisis gets a bad reputation, painted as a millennial indulgence or a failure to launch. The truth is far more interesting: this period of upheaval represents a critical phase in adult development, as natural and necessary as the awkwardness of adolescence[14].

During this phase, your brain is conducting a massive integration project. The prefrontal cortex, finally reaching full development, is trying to reconcile who you thought you'd become with who you're actually becoming. The schemas you developed in childhood are meeting the realities of adult life, and often, they don't match[15].

David's experience illustrates this integration challenge perfectly. At twenty-six, he was on his fourth job in three years, each transition marked by the same pattern. He'd start with enthusiasm, throw himself into the work, then gradually feel a creeping sense of emptiness. His "unrelenting standards" schema demanded perfection, but perfection in service of what? His parents had clear visions for his career—doctor, lawyer, engineer. David had dutifully tried variations of each, excelling at all and enjoying none.

The crisis came when David realized he was living someone else's definition of success. The achievements that were supposed to bring satisfaction brought only exhaustion. His LinkedIn looked impressive, but his life felt hollow. The cocoon phase began when he finally asked: "What do I actually want?"

The Identity Puzzle: Building Yourself from Scratch

Young adulthood presents a unique challenge: you're expected to know who you are while you're still figuring it out. Unlike previous generations who often had clearer scripts—work at the company, marry by twenty-five, buy the house—today's young adults face infinite options and fewer clear pathways[16].

This abundance of choice can paradoxically make identity formation harder. When you can be anything, how do you choose to be something specific? The schemas that once provided direction ("I'm the smart one," "I'm the helper," "I'm the rebel") may no longer fit the complex adult you're becoming.

Emma faced this puzzle at twenty-four. Known in her family as "the responsible one," she'd built her identity around being reliable, predictable, safe. Her career in accounting fit perfectly—stable, respectable, clear advancement path. But Emma had a secret: she spent her evenings writing comedy sketches and performing at open mics under a stage name.

The cognitive dissonance was exhausting. Responsible Emma wore blazers and analyzed spreadsheets. Secret Emma told jokes about existential dread to strangers in basements. For months, she maintained both identities, feeling like a fraud in each. The crisis peaked when her company offered a promotion that would lock her into the accounting track for years. Emma had to decide: which version of herself was real?

Decision-Making in the Fog of Not Knowing

The quarter-life crisis is characterized by a particular kind of decision paralysis. Unlike the concrete choices of earlier life stages—which college to attend, which major to choose—young adult decisions feel both more consequential and more ambiguous.

Should you take the stable job or the risky opportunity? Stay in your hometown or move across the country? Invest in graduate school or gain work experience? Each choice feels like it's determining your entire future, yet you lack the life experience to predict outcomes accurately.

Alex exemplified this paralysis. At twenty-five, he had three job offers: a corporate position with excellent benefits, a startup role with equity potential, and a nonprofit job aligned with his values but paying half as much. He created spreadsheets, consulted mentors, made pro-con lists that went on for pages. Six weeks later, he'd lost all three opportunities to his indecision.

What Alex didn't understand was that his "failure" schema was sabotaging his decision-making process. Deep down, he believed any choice would be wrong because he was fundamentally inadequate. No amount of analysis could overcome this core belief. The fog wasn't from lack of information—it was from schema-driven fear.

The Comparison Trap 2.0: Social Media and Life Timelines

If regular social media comparison is difficult, quarter-life crisis comparison is brutal. Your feed becomes a highlight reel of others hitting traditional milestones: engagements, mortgages, babies, promotions. Each announcement can feel like evidence that you're falling behind in a race you didn't sign up for.

The comparison trap during quarter-life crisis has a particular sting because it plays directly into schemas of inadequacy and failure. When you're already questioning your direction, seeing others' apparent certainty feels like confirmation that something's wrong with you.

Emma's Instagram feed became a source of daily torment. High school classmates posted engagement photos in apple orchards. College friends shared home renovation projects. Her cousin, two years younger, announced her pregnancy with a photoshoot that probably cost more than Emma's monthly rent. Each post felt like a referendum on Emma's life choices.

What Emma couldn't see through the schema fog was that many of those posting were running their own races with their own doubts. The friend with the perfect engagement photos would confide months later about relationship anxiety. The cousin with the baby would admit to feeling like she'd lost herself in motherhood. Instagram didn't show the full story—it never does.

Building Your Identity GPS: Values, Strengths, and Direction

The path through quarter-life crisis isn't about finding the right answer—it's about developing your own navigation system. This involves three key components: clarifying your values, recognizing your strengths, and accepting that direction emerges through movement, not contemplation.

Values clarification sounds simple but proves challenging when you've been living by inherited values. David discovered this when he finally stopped running from job to job and asked himself what mattered. His parents valued prestige and financial security. His peers valued innovation and disruption. But what did David value?

Through systematic exploration—journaling, therapy, long conversations with trusted friends—David identified his core values: creativity, connection, and contribution. These had been present all along, suppressed by his unrelenting standards schema that prioritized external achievement over internal alignment. Once clear on his values, decisions became easier. He chose work that might look less impressive on paper but felt authentic to who he was becoming.

Recognizing strengths requires separating what you're good at from what others have praised you for. Emma was excellent at accounting—detail-oriented, systematic, reliable. But these strengths weren't limited to spreadsheets. Her comedy succeeded because she brought the same precision to timing, the same attention to structure, the same reliability to showing up and practicing.

The revelation came when Emma stopped seeing her identities as opposing forces. The responsible one and the comedian weren't different people—they were different expressions of the same strengths. This integration allowed her to create a life that honored both aspects, keeping her day job while building her comedy career, eventually transitioning when the balance felt right.

Direction emerges through experimentation, not revelation. Alex learned this after his paralysis cost him three opportunities. Instead of waiting for certainty, he began taking small steps in different directions. He volunteered with the nonprofit on weekends. He did contract work for the startup. He attended corporate networking events. Through action rather than analysis, patterns emerged. He discovered he valued mission over money but needed some financial stability to feel secure. This led to choices that honored both needs.

Navigating Your Quarter-Life Crisis: A Practical Guide

Understanding the quarter-life crisis as a developmental phase rather than a personal failure changes everything. Here are strategies for moving through this transition with greater ease and self-compassion:

Values Archaeology Exercise: Spend a week noticing what genuinely energizes you versus what drains you. Pay attention to moments of authentic excitement or deep satisfaction. These emotional responses point toward your true values, often buried under layers of "should."

The Three Lives Exercise: Imagine you could live three completely different lives. What would they be? A artist in Berlin? A teacher in your hometown? A entrepreneur in Silicon Valley? Write out each life in detail. Notice which elements appear across all three—these point to core desires that can be honored in multiple ways.

Quarter-Life Crisis Reframe: Instead of "I'm behind," try "I'm becoming." Instead of "Everyone else knows what they're doing," try "Everyone is figuring it out." Instead of "I should have it together by now," try "Development takes time." These reframes honor the process rather than rushing toward an imaginary finish line.

Decision Momentum Practice: When facing a decision, set a deadline. Make the best choice you can with available information, then commit to learning from the outcome. Remember: most young adult decisions are reversible. The cost of indecision often exceeds the cost of a imperfect choice.

Comparison Detox Protocol: For one month, when you notice comparison arising, immediately do three things: name what schema is activated, identify one thing you're grateful for in your own life, and reach out to support someone else. This interrupts the comparison neural pathway and builds new patterns of gratitude and connection.

The quarter-life crisis isn't a problem to be solved but a chrysalis to be honored. The confusion, doubt, and searching aren't signs of failure—they're signs of growth. Your brain is doing exactly what it's supposed to do: questioning inherited patterns, exploring possibilities, and gradually constructing an identity that's authentically yours.

The discomfort means you're alive to your own becoming. Trust the process, even when—especially when—you can't see where it leads.

Key Takeaways

- The quarter-life crisis represents a necessary developmental phase where your brain integrates childhood schemas with adult realities, creating temporary but important instability

- Identity confusion during this period is normal and healthy—you're building yourself from scratch rather than following predetermined scripts

- Decision paralysis often stems from underlying schemas of failure or inadequacy rather than lack of information or options

- Social media comparison during quarter-life crisis particularly stings because it reinforces schemas while showing only curated success stories

- Building your own navigation system through values clarification, strength recognition, and experimental action provides direction more effectively than endless analysis

Chapter 4: Dating Your Schemas - Relationship Pattern Recognition

The swipe comes so naturally now. Left for no, right for maybe, the endless scroll of faces becoming a blur of possibility and disappointment. But what if the real pattern isn't in who you're swiping on, but in what drives the swipe itself? Your dating life isn't just about finding the right person—it's about understanding the invisible blueprint that guides every romantic choice you make.

Your Love Blueprint - How Family Scripts Show Up on Dating Apps

Every dating profile you create, every message you send, every person you find attractive carries the fingerprints of your earliest experiences with love. The family you grew up in wrote the first draft of your relationship script, and now you're living it out one swipe at a time[17].

Maya discovered this at twenty-six when she noticed a disturbing pattern. Every man she dated seriously was some variation of emotionally unavailable. There was James, who could only express feelings after three drinks. Marcus, who responded to "I love you" with "Thanks." Dev, who disappeared for days when conversations got too real. At first, Maya blamed bad luck or the modern dating pool. Then she started connecting dots.

Growing up, Maya's father was physically present but emotionally absent. He provided well, showed up to school events, but never quite seemed to see her. Love meant being chosen by someone just out of reach. Now, on dating apps, she unconsciously screened for the familiar—men whose profiles hinted at distance, whose communication style felt slightly cold, whose availability seemed conditional.

The blueprint revealed itself in her swiping patterns. Profiles with emotional availability—"Looking for something real," "Ready to build something together"—triggered immediate left swipes. Too needy, she'd think. Too intense. But profiles with subtle red flags—"Not sure what I'm looking for," "Just seeing what's out there"—sparked intrigue. The challenge activated something deep in her nervous system, a familiar dance of pursuing the unpursuable.

Your family-of-origin patterns don't just influence who you choose; they determine what feels like chemistry. That spark you feel might actually be your nervous system recognizing a familiar dysfunction. The person who makes your heart race might be activating old wounds rather than genuine connection.

The Attachment Style Dating Game - Secure, Anxious, or Avoidant?

Attachment theory has become dating vocabulary, with people listing their style like astrological signs. But understanding your attachment pattern goes deeper than pop psychology labels—it's about recognizing how early relationships created a template for all future connections[18].

Jake exemplified the avoidant attachment style in action. His dating profile was a masterclass in mixed signals: great photos suggesting availability, bio full of humor but no real personal information, "looking for something casual, but open to more with the right person." Translation: I want connection but on my terms, at my pace, with multiple exit routes.

His pattern was predictable. First dates went brilliantly—he was charming, attentive, genuinely interested. Second and third dates maintained the momentum. But somewhere around date five or six, when things started feeling real, Jake would feel an overwhelming urge to run. His body would literally rebel—tightness in chest, urge to flee, sudden awareness of every flaw in his date.

Jake had mastered what he called "ethical ghosting." He'd send a thoughtful message about not being ready, wishing them the best, then disappear completely. No social media connections, no chance encounters, no possibility of reconnection. Clean breaks, he reasoned, were kinder. What he didn't realize was that his avoidant attachment wasn't protecting anyone—it was preventing him from experiencing the very connection he claimed to want.

Sarah represented the anxious attachment style. Where Jake fled from connection, Sarah clung to it. Her phone became command central for relationship anxiety. She analyzed response times (why did he take three hours to reply?), decoded emoji usage (what did that single heart mean versus double hearts?), and created elaborate theories about digital behavior.

Sarah's text anxiety wasn't really about texts. Growing up with an inconsistent mother—loving one day, distant the next—she'd learned that love required constant vigilance. You had to monitor for signs of withdrawal, work to maintain connection, never relax into security. Now, at twenty-four, she brought that same hypervigilance to dating. Every delayed response triggered abandonment fears. Every moment of distance felt like impending loss.

The cruel irony? Sarah's anxious behavior often created the very abandonment she feared. Her need for constant reassurance exhausted partners. Her emotional intensity in early dating stages scared off potential matches. Her anxiety became a self-fulfilling prophecy, confirming her core belief that love always leaves.

Red Flags or Schema Triggers? Decoding Your Dating Reactions

Not every strong reaction in dating signals a red flag. Sometimes, what feels like intuition is actually a schema being triggered. Learning to differentiate between genuine warning signs and your own psychological patterns can revolutionize your dating life.

Consider the difference: A red flag is behavior that indicates potential harm—lying, disrespect, boundary violations. A schema trigger is a neutral behavior that activates your old wounds—someone needing space (triggering abandonment fears), someone being confident (triggering defectiveness beliefs), someone showing interest (triggering mistrust schemas).

Maya experienced this confusion constantly. When a date showed genuine interest—texting regularly, making plans, expressing feelings—her mistrust schema activated. "What does he want?" her mind would race. "What's his angle?" She'd interpret normal courtship behavior as manipulation, creating distance to protect herself from imagined threats.

Jake's schema triggers were more subtle. Whenever someone wanted to leave belongings at his apartment—a toothbrush, a sweater—his enmeshment schema activated. Those objects felt like invasion, like loss of self. A simple toothbrush became symbolic of his entire identity being swallowed by relationship. His strong reaction wasn't about dental hygiene; it was about a childhood where boundaries didn't exist.

Sarah's triggers centered around communication gaps. If someone didn't respond immediately, her abandonment schema created catastrophic narratives. He's with someone else. He's realized I'm not worth it. He's planning how to leave. The reality—he was in a meeting, his phone died, he was driving—couldn't compete with schema-driven storytelling.

Breaking the Cycle - From Unconscious Patterns to Conscious Choices

Recognition is the first step, but breaking patterns requires deliberate practice. The goal isn't to eliminate all emotional responses but to create space between trigger and reaction, between feeling and behavior[19].

Maya began with what she called "pause practice." When she felt attracted to someone, she'd pause and ask: "What feels familiar about this person?" If the answer involved distance, unavailability, or challenge, she'd flag it as pattern rather than preference. This didn't mean automatic rejection, but it meant proceeding with awareness.

She also started experimenting with dating against type. She forced herself to go on three dates with anyone who seemed "too available" or "too nice." The experiment revealed something shocking: her nervous system could adapt. What initially felt boring gradually became comfortable. What seemed like lack of chemistry was actually absence of anxiety.

Jake's pattern-breaking involved gradual exposure to intimacy. He started small—leaving his own belongings at his apartment in visible places when dates came over. Then allowing someone to leave a phone charger. Then a book. Each step challenged his enmeshment fears without overwhelming his system. He learned that connection didn't mean consumption, that you could be close without losing yourself.

His biggest breakthrough came when he started sharing his pattern with dates. "I have avoidant attachment," he'd explain. "Around date five or six, I might feel like running. It's not about you—it's my pattern. I'm working on it." This transparency changed everything. Partners could support rather than chase. His urge to flee decreased when it wasn't a secret.

Building Secure Love - Relationship Skills for the Digital Age

Secure attachment isn't just for the lucky few who had perfect childhoods. It's a learnable skill set that can be developed through conscious practice and safe relationships[20]. The digital age presents unique challenges but also opportunities for practicing security.

First, understand that dating apps aren't the enemy. They're tools that amplify existing patterns. If you have anxious attachment, apps provide endless opportunities for rejection sensitivity. If you're avoidant, they offer infinite escape routes. But they also allow unprecedented control over pace and exposure to different relationship styles.

Building security starts with regulating your own nervous system. Before swiping, before dates, before difficult conversations, check in with your body. Are you activated? Anxious? Shut down? Simple breathing exercises, movement, or grounding techniques can shift you from reactive to responsive.

Sarah developed a pre-date ritual: five minutes of meditation, writing three things she appreciated about herself, setting an intention for curiosity rather than outcome. This practice helped her show up as herself rather than her anxiety. She learned to treat dates as experiments in connection rather than auditions for love.

Communication in the digital age requires new skills. Texting removes tone, body language, and immediate feedback—all crucial for secure attachment. The solution isn't avoiding digital communication but being intentional about it. Clear, direct messages reduce anxiety for everyone. "I'm interested in seeing you again" beats subtle hints. "I need some time to process" beats unexplained silence.

Practical Tools for Schema-Aware Dating

Dating with schema awareness doesn't mean analyzing every interaction or pathologizing every feeling. It means bringing consciousness to patterns that usually run unconsciously. Here are practical tools for navigating modern dating with greater awareness:

The Dating Schema Detective Worksheet: Track patterns across multiple dates. Notice who you're attracted to, what triggers anxiety or excitement, when you want to pursue or flee. Look for themes rather than judging individual experiences.

Family Love Map Exercise: Draw your family tree but instead of names, write relationship patterns. How did people show love? Handle conflict? Deal with intimacy? Notice which patterns you're repeating or rebelling against.

Schema-Aware Dating Profile Creation: Write your profile from your healthiest self, not your schemas. If you're anxiously attached, resist overexplaining or people-pleasing. If you're avoidant, include some genuine vulnerability. Let your profile attract people who appreciate your authentic self.

Trigger Response Planning: Identify your top three dating triggers and create planned responses. If abandonment fears spike with delayed texts, plan to: breathe, remind yourself of alternative explanations, engage in self-soothing activity, respond when calm. Having a plan reduces reactive behavior.

Secure Communication Scripts: Develop go-to phrases for common situations. "I'm feeling activated and need a moment to ground myself." "I notice I'm making up stories about what this means—can you help me understand?" "I care about you and also need to maintain my own boundaries."

The journey from schema-driven dating to conscious relationship building isn't about finding someone without issues—everyone has patterns. It's about developing enough awareness to choose partners whose patterns complement rather than trigger yours, and enough skills to work through activation together. Your dating life can become a laboratory for growth rather than a repetition of old wounds. The patterns that once controlled you can become information that guides you toward healthier love.

Bridge to Growth

As you begin recognizing these patterns in your romantic life, you might notice similar dynamics playing out in another arena—your career. The same schemas that influence who you're attracted to also shape how you show up at work, particularly around feelings of competence and belonging. The impostor syndrome so common among young professionals isn't just about career insecurity; it's often the workplace expression of the same core schemas affecting your relationships.

Key Takeaways

- Your dating patterns directly reflect early attachment experiences and family dynamics, with attraction often signaling familiar dysfunction rather than genuine compatibility

- Attachment styles (secure, anxious, avoidant) create predictable patterns in digital dating behavior that can be recognized and modified through conscious practice

- Strong emotional reactions in dating may be schema triggers rather than intuition—learning to differentiate helps you make choices based on present reality rather than past wounds

- Breaking unconscious patterns requires deliberate practice including dating against type, transparency about attachment style, and gradual exposure to healthy intimacy

- Secure attachment is a learnable skill that can be developed through nervous system regulation, clear communication, and schema-aware dating practices

Chapter 5: The Impostor Syndrome Solution - Career and Achievement Fears

The email sits in your drafts folder for the third day. It's a simple request for a raise, backed by solid performance metrics, but you can't hit send. The voice in your head is louder than logic: "They'll realize you don't deserve what you're already making. They'll see through the facade. They'll discover you've been faking competence this whole time." This is impostor syndrome speaking, and for young adults entering today's workforce, it's reached epidemic proportions[21].

Generation Fake It - Why Young Adults Feel Like Career Frauds

The modern workplace creates perfect conditions for impostor syndrome to flourish. Social media broadcasts everyone's wins while hiding their struggles. LinkedIn feeds overflow with promotions, launches, and humble brags. Entry-level jobs demand five years of experience. The gig economy promises freedom but delivers instability. No wonder young professionals feel like they're performing competence rather than possessing it.

Jennifer's story captures this generational struggle. At twenty-seven, she was a marketing manager at a tech startup, managing million-dollar campaigns and a team of five. Her performance reviews consistently exceeded expectations. Clients requested her specifically. Yet every morning, Jennifer woke with the same thought: "Today's the day they figure out I have no idea what I'm doing."

The evidence of her competence couldn't penetrate the fog of her fraudulence schema. She attributed every success to luck, timing, or team effort—never to her own abilities. When praised, she deflected. When promoted, she panicked. The higher she climbed, the farther she felt she had to fall when inevitably "exposed."

Jennifer's impostor syndrome had a particular modern twist. She'd learned her job largely through YouTube tutorials, online courses, and trial and error—not formal education. In her mind, this made her knowledge less legitimate than someone with an MBA. She didn't realize that her self-directed learning demonstrated exactly the adaptability and initiative employers valued most.

The Schema Behind the Syndrome - Understanding Your Achievement Fears

Impostor syndrome isn't a character flaw or millennial weakness—it's typically a manifestation of deeper schemas formed in childhood[22]. The most common culprits include the defectiveness schema ("I'm fundamentally flawed"), the failure schema ("I'm destined to fail"), and the unrelenting standards schema ("Nothing I do is ever good enough").

David exemplified how unrelenting standards create impostor feelings. Growing up in a high-achieving family where B+ meant failure, he'd internalized impossible benchmarks for success. Now, at twenty-nine, he worked seventy-hour weeks as a consultant, triple-checking every deliverable, staying late to perfect presentations that were already excellent.

The cruel irony? His perfectionism made him feel more fraudulent, not less. He reasoned that if he had real talent, work wouldn't require such effort. True experts, he believed, found things easy. His schema blinded him to the reality that expertise comes through effort, not despite it.

David's impostor syndrome manifested in specific workplace behaviors. He never took credit in meetings, always deflecting to team effort. He over-prepared for everything, creating forty-slide decks when ten would suffice. He avoided visibility, turning down speaking opportunities and high-profile projects. Each avoidance reinforced his core belief: "If they really knew me, they'd see I'm not as capable as they think."

Kai represented a different schema expression. Her subjugation schema—developed in a family where her needs always came last—created impostor syndrome through different mechanisms. She felt fraudulent not because she lacked skills, but because she couldn't advocate for herself. Taking up space, asking for resources, setting boundaries all felt like playing a character rather than being herself.

Millennial Mind Games - Navigating Workplace Dynamics

The generational divide in workplace expectations adds another layer to impostor syndrome. Young adults often find themselves caught between old-school hierarchy and new-world flexibility, trying to decode unwritten rules while pretending they already understand them[23].

Kai's relationship with her Gen X boss illustrated this perfectly. Her manager valued face time, believing real work happened in offices between nine and five. Kai, who did her best thinking at home in evening hours, felt constantly judged for her work style. She started arriving early and staying late—not to work, but to be seen working. This performance of productivity made her feel even more fraudulent.

The feedback disconnect worsened her impostor syndrome. Her boss gave feedback annually in formal reviews. Kai, raised on instant digital feedback, interpreted the silence between reviews as evidence of inadequacy. She created elaborate narratives about what the absence of praise meant, each day without feedback confirming her fraudulence fears.

Different generational approaches to boundaries created additional challenges. When Kai tried setting healthy work-life boundaries—not checking email after 8 PM, taking actual lunch breaks—she worried about being seen as uncommitted compared to older colleagues who wore burnout like badges of honor. She felt like an impostor for prioritizing sustainability over sacrifice.

From Comparison to Confidence - Social Media and Career FOMO

Professional social media platforms have transformed career comparison from occasional to constant. Every scroll through LinkedIn presents evidence of others' success, triggering schemas around inadequacy and failure. The platform's algorithm ensures you see the wins—the promotions, the speaking engagements, the thought leadership—while hiding the struggles.

Jennifer found herself in a toxic cycle with LinkedIn. She'd post about work achievements to combat impostor feelings, then feel fraudulent about the positive responses. The likes and congratulations felt hollow because they responded to her curated professional image, not her inner experience of inadequacy. Each post deepened the gap between external perception and internal reality.

The comparison trap hit hardest with peers from college. Watching classmates announce exciting ventures while she sat in corporate meetings made Jennifer question every career choice. She didn't see their student loans, their sixty-hour weeks, their own impostor struggles. Social media showed only outcomes, not process.

Breaking free required radical honesty. Jennifer started sharing not just wins but challenges. She posted about projects that failed, lessons learned from mistakes, moments of professional doubt. The response surprised her—vulnerability created deeper connections than success stories. Other young professionals messaged privately, sharing their own impostor experiences. The fraudulence felt less isolating when she realized its universality.

Authentic Achievement - Building Real Confidence

The solution to impostor syndrome isn't more achievement—it's changing your relationship with achievement itself. This means recognizing that competence and confidence develop through practice, not perfection. It means valuing growth over performance, process over outcome[24].

David's breakthrough came through what he called "competence mapping." He listed every skill required for his job, then rated his ability in each from 1-10. The exercise revealed something shocking: he was highly competent in most areas, developing in others, and weak in only a few. His impostor syndrome had created a global sense of inadequacy from limited areas of growth.

He then tracked how these ratings changed over six months. Watching his competence grow through effort and experience challenged his fixed mindset about ability. Skills he'd struggled with became strengths. New challenges emerged as others were mastered. Competence wasn't a state to achieve but a process to engage.

Jennifer addressed her fraudulence schema through "evidence collection." Every day, she wrote down three pieces of evidence of her competence—problems solved, value added, skills demonstrated. At first, her schema fought back, minimizing each accomplishment. But the daily practice gradually built a database her impostor syndrome couldn't argue with.

The evidence collection evolved into what she called "impact tracking." Instead of focusing on her perceived competence, she tracked her actual impact—campaigns that drove results, team members who grew under her leadership, clients who renewed contracts. Impact was harder for her schema to dismiss than subjective self-assessment.

Practical Strategies for Schema-Informed Professional Development

Addressing impostor syndrome requires both internal work on schemas and external changes in how you approach professional life. Here are evidence-based strategies for building authentic confidence:

Success Evidence Journal: Each day, document three professional wins, no matter how small. Include not just what you achieved but how you achieved it. This builds a concrete record your impostor syndrome can't erase.

Schema Dialogue Practice: When impostor thoughts arise, engage them directly. "I hear you saying I'm not qualified. What evidence supports that? What evidence challenges it?" Treat impostor thoughts as outdated protection rather than truth.

Values-Based Career Mapping: Define success by your values, not external metrics. If growth matters more than position, measure learning rather than promotions. If impact matters more than income, track contribution rather than salary. Aligned metrics reduce impostor feelings.

Mistake Reframing Ritual: When you make errors (inevitable in any career), practice immediate reframing. "This mistake teaches me X." "This failure provides data about Y." "This challenge develops skill Z." Mistakes become curriculum rather than evidence of fraudulence.

Vulnerable Leadership Experiments: Share one professional struggle or learning edge with colleagues weekly. Notice how vulnerability creates connection rather than judgment. Leadership includes acknowledging growth areas, not just showcasing strengths.

The journey from impostor syndrome to authentic confidence isn't about finally feeling adequate—it's about acting with purpose despite inadequacy feelings. Your schemas may never fully disappear, but they can transform from controllers to informants. The voice saying "you're not enough" becomes just one perspective among many, no longer the director of your professional life.

Moving Forward Together

As you develop awareness of how schemas shape your professional life, you might notice similar patterns emerging in another crucial area—your friendships. The same core beliefs that create impostor syndrome at work often dictate how you show up in social relationships. The roles you play, the boundaries you set (or don't), and the connections you create all reflect the deeper patterns we're learning to recognize and reshape.

Key Takeaways

- Impostor syndrome represents schemas playing out in professional contexts, with childhood patterns of defectiveness, failure, or unrelenting standards manifesting as career fraudulence fears

- Generational workplace differences intensify impostor feelings as young adults navigate between traditional hierarchies and modern flexibility while pretending to understand unwritten rules

- Professional social media amplifies impostor syndrome through constant success comparison, showing only curated wins while hiding universal struggles

- Building authentic confidence requires shifting from performance to growth mindset, collecting evidence of competence, and aligning success metrics with personal values rather than external expectations

- Vulnerability and transparency about professional challenges create deeper connections and reduce impostor isolation more effectively than projecting false confidence

Chapter 6: Family Patterns in Adult Friendships - Social Dynamics

The dinner invitation triggers familiar dread. Your friends want to celebrate someone's promotion, but you know how it will go. You'll arrive early to help set up, stay late to clean, spend the evening making sure everyone else is comfortable while your own needs remain unspoken. By the time you get home, exhausted and somehow lonely despite being surrounded by people, you'll wonder why friendship feels so much like work. What you might not realize is that you're not just attending a dinner party—you're reenacting your childhood role in every social situation.

Your Family's Friendship Blueprint

The first social system you ever knew was your family. Before you learned about friendship, you learned about relationships through parents, siblings, and extended family dynamics. These early experiences created a blueprint that now unconsciously guides how you form and maintain adult friendships[25].

Lisa discovered this connection at twenty-eight when she found herself exhausted by a friend group she supposedly loved. Growing up as the eldest of four with overwhelmed parents, she'd been the family caretaker since age ten— making lunches, helping with homework, mediating sibling fights. Love meant being useful. Worth came through service.

Now, her adult friendships followed the same script. Lisa was the friend everyone called in crisis but no one checked on. She organized birthday parties, remembered important dates, offered free therapy sessions over wine. Her friends loved her, but they loved what she did for them more than who she was. The pattern was so familiar she didn't recognize it as a pattern—just as how friendship worked.

The blueprint revealed itself in specific behaviors. When friends gathered, Lisa automatically scanned for needs: Who looked sad? Who needed a drink refill? Who was standing alone? She couldn't relax into just being present. Her nervous system, trained through years of family vigilance, stayed on high alert for problems to solve, people to care for, harmony to maintain.

Mike's blueprint operated differently. In his family, connection happened through screens. His parents, both remote workers, showed love through shared digital experiences—gaming together, sending memes, family group chats. Physical presence felt uncomfortable; digital interaction felt safe. Now at twenty-five, Mike had dozens of online friendships but struggled with in-person connection.

His social anxiety wasn't just introversion—it was a schema-driven response to unfamiliar territory. Real-world friendship required skills his family never modeled: reading body language, navigating physical space, tolerating awkward silences. Online, he was witty and engaged. In person, he felt like an actor forgetting his lines.

Social Anxiety in the Digital Age

Social anxiety among young adults has reached unprecedented levels, and it's not just about being shy[26]. The intersection of schemas, digital communication, and reduced in-person interaction during formative years creates perfect conditions for social fears to flourish.

Taylor's emotional inhibition schema turned every social interaction into a performance. Growing up in a family where emotions were "drama" and vulnerability was weakness, they'd learned to present a carefully controlled version of themselves. Now at twenty-three, maintaining this facade across multiple friend groups felt impossible.

The digital age complicated Taylor's schema. Online, they could craft perfect responses, edit out awkwardness, present their ideal self. In-person gatherings removed these controls. Without time to compose thoughts, filter reactions, or manage impressions, Taylor felt exposed. Their solution? Avoid in-person gatherings whenever possible, maintaining friendships through carefully curated digital interactions.

But digital friendship came with its own anxieties. Group chats moved too fast to craft perfect responses. Video calls removed the safety of invisibility. Even Instagram stories felt risky—what if the real Taylor showed through? The emotional inhibition that once protected them in family dynamics now imprisoned them in adult friendships.

Social media adds another layer of complexity. Watching friends post group photos from gatherings you weren't invited to triggers abandonment schemas. Seeing others' seemingly effortless social lives activates defectiveness beliefs. The constant performance of friendship online exhausts those already struggling with connection.

The Friendship Roles We Play - People-Pleaser, Rescuer, or Invisible?

Just as families have roles—the responsible one, the rebel, the peacemaker—adult friend groups often recreate these dynamics. Without awareness, you might find yourself playing the same character in every social setting, wondering why different friend groups feel remarkably similar[27].

Lisa perfected the rescuer role across multiple contexts. In her work friend group, she mediated conflicts. Among college friends, she provided free counseling. With neighbors, she became the emergency contact. Each group saw her as endlessly capable and giving, not recognizing her caretaking as a compulsion rather than choice.

The rescuer role provided secondary benefits that made it hard to abandon. People needed her, which felt like love. Crises gave her purpose. Others' problems distracted from her own unmet needs. But the cost was steep: chronic exhaustion, resentment toward friends who took without giving, and deep loneliness despite constant company.

Mike played the invisible friend—present but not really there. In group settings, he positioned himself physically at edges, psychologically at margins. He laughed at others' jokes without making his own, asked questions without sharing answers, attended events without fully participating. His withdrawal schema made real connection feel dangerous.

The invisible role felt safe but created its own pain. Friends forgot to invite him places, assuming he wouldn't come. They shared surface-level chat but no real intimacy. Mike wanted deeper friendships but couldn't risk the visibility required to create them. His schema kept him trapped in the periphery of every social circle.

Taylor embodied the people-pleaser, shapeshifting based on who they were with. With artistic friends, they emphasized their creative side. With athletic friends, they talked fitness.

With political friends, they matched the expected ideology. This constant adaptation exhausted them, and worse, left them feeling unknown by anyone.

Breaking Free from Social Scripts

Recognizing your friendship patterns is the first step toward changing them. But recognition alone isn't enough—you need practical strategies for showing up differently in social situations where schemas run strong.

Lisa began by implementing what she called "conscious non-helping." At social gatherings, she gave herself permission to not solve problems, not caretake, not manage others' emotions. The first attempts were agonizing. Watching a friend struggle without intervening triggered every alarm in her nervous system. Her schema screamed that she was being selfish, unloving, bad.

But something interesting happened. Without Lisa jumping in to fix everything, her friends started solving their own problems. They began checking on her, noticing when she seemed tired or stressed. The friendships didn't fall apart without her caretaking—they became more reciprocal. Her friends had been willing to show up for her all along; her rescuing had prevented them from trying.

Mike challenged his invisible role through "visibility practice." He started small—sharing one personal story per social gathering, stating one preference when groups made plans, expressing one opinion during discussions. Each visibility moment terrified him, but also created connection. Friends responded with curiosity about this newly emerging Mike.

His biggest breakthrough came when he hosted a gathering himself. Having control over the environment—his space, his

47

guest list, his activity choice—made visibility feel safer. Friends saw his apartment, met his cat, experienced his hospitality. The host role forced him out of the margins into the center, revealing that visibility didn't lead to rejection but to deeper connection.

Building Your Chosen Family

The beauty of adult friendship is choice. Unlike family relationships, you can consciously create a social network that supports your growth rather than reinforces your schemas. This requires intention, boundaries, and willingness to release relationships that keep you stuck in old patterns[28].

Taylor's friendship revolution began with an audit. They listed all their friendships and honestly assessed which ones required performance versus allowed authenticity. The results were stark—most relationships demanded they be someone they weren't. Taylor made the difficult decision to invest less in performance-based friendships and seek connections that welcomed their full self.

Finding schema-aware friends required vulnerability. Taylor started being honest about their struggles with emotional expression, their family background, their desire for deeper connection. This honesty filtered out those who wanted only surface interaction while attracting others on similar growth journeys. Slowly, Taylor built a chosen family of friends who celebrated rather than feared emotional authenticity.

Lisa learned to recognize potential friends who wouldn't activate her caretaking schema. She looked for people with their own support systems, who offered help as often as they accepted it, who noticed and respected her boundaries.

These friendships felt foreign at first—what do you do with friends who don't need rescuing? Gradually, Lisa discovered: you enjoy them.

Creating Schema-Informed Friendships: Practical Strategies

Building healthier friendships while healing schemas requires both internal work and external changes. Here are concrete strategies for transforming your social life:

Friendship Pattern Mapping: Create a visual map of your friendships, noting which role you play in each. Look for patterns across different groups. Are you always the helper? The entertainer? The advice-giver? Recognition precedes change.

Friendship Archaeology: Explore how your current friendships mirror family dynamics. Which friends remind you of family members? Which interactions feel familiar from childhood? Understanding these parallels helps you choose differently.

Authentic Sharing Practice: In safe friendships, practice sharing one authentic thing weekly—a real feeling, a genuine struggle, an unpopular opinion. Notice how vulnerability deepens connection rather than destroying it.

Social Boundary Setting: Identify one boundary you need in friendships (saying no to favors, limiting advice-giving, protecting alone time). Practice stating this boundary clearly and maintaining it despite discomfort.

Schema-Aware Friend Selection: When meeting new people, notice schema activation. Do they trigger caretaking? Performance anxiety? Invisibility urges? Use this information to choose friends who support your growth rather than reinforce patterns.

The transformation from schema-driven to conscious friendship doesn't happen overnight. You'll find yourself falling into old roles, especially during stress. But each moment of awareness, each different choice, each authentic interaction rewires your social blueprint. The friends who can't handle your growth will fade; those who celebrate it will emerge. Your social life becomes a laboratory for practicing new ways of being, surrounded by chosen family who see and support your true self.

Looking Back to Move Forward

The patterns we've explored—in relationships, career, and friendships—all point to a deeper truth: money and self-worth are intimately connected in ways our schemas determine. As we prepare to examine how these same patterns influence financial behavior, consider how the roles you play in friendships might mirror the story you tell yourself about deserving abundance or struggling with scarcity.

Key Takeaways

- Adult friendships unconsciously recreate family dynamics, with early relationship blueprints determining how you form and maintain social connections

- Digital age social anxiety stems from schemas interacting with reduced in-person practice and the pressure of curated online personas

- Friend groups recreate family roles—rescuer, people-pleaser, invisible one—keeping you trapped in familiar but limiting patterns

- Breaking free requires conscious visibility practice, boundary setting, and releasing performance-based friendships that reinforce schemas

- Building chosen family means selecting friends who support growth rather than activate old patterns, creating space for authentic connection

Chapter 7: Money, Success, and Self-Worth - Financial Behavior Patterns

The notification pings at 2 AM. Your credit card payment is due tomorrow, and you're lying awake calculating if you can make minimum payment while still affording groceries. The shame feels physical—a weight on your chest, heat in your face. You know you shouldn't have bought those concert tickets, that dinner out, that online course promising to change your life. But somehow, in the moment, each purchase felt necessary, even inevitable. This isn't just about money. It's about the story you tell yourself about what you deserve, what you're worth, and what love looks like with a price tag attached.

The Money Story You Tell Yourself

Every financial decision you make is filtered through a narrative written long before you earned your first paycheck. This money story—assembled from family messages, cultural beliefs, and early experiences—operates like an invisible script directing your financial behavior[29].

Maya's story began in a middle-class household where money was simultaneously scarce and secret. Her parents maintained appearances—nice clothes, newer cars, the right neighborhood—while fighting behind closed doors about credit card bills. Love looked like material provision. Stress smelled like final notices hidden in drawers. Success meant looking like you had more than you did.

Now at twenty-five, Maya lived her own version of this story. Her Instagram showcased brunches at trendy restaurants, weekend trips, a carefully curated apartment. Behind the camera, she juggled six credit cards, paid overdraft fees monthly, and felt physically sick checking her bank balance. The pattern was so familiar she didn't recognize it as learned behavior—just how life worked.

Maya's money story had specific chapters: "People who love you buy you things" (so she overspent on friends). "Your worth shows in what you own" (so she accumulated designer items she couldn't afford). "Money problems should be hidden" (so she never asked for help). Each belief drove behaviors that deepened her financial stress while feeling completely logical from inside her story.

David told himself a different tale. Growing up in an affluent family where money was plentiful but conditional, he learned that financial success was the entry fee for belonging. His father, a successful surgeon, made it clear: achievement brought approval, failure brought disappointment. Money wasn't just currency—it was the scoreboard of human value.

Despite earning good money as a software engineer, David lived in constant financial anxiety. He checked his accounts obsessively, tracking every penny like his worthiness depended on it (because in his story, it did). He couldn't enjoy what he had, always focused on not having enough. The number needed for "enough" kept moving—first 50K savings, then 100K, then a million. No amount could fill the hole where self-worth should be.

When Your Bank Account Becomes Your Scorecard

The conflation of net worth with self-worth has reached new extremes in the social media age. Financial success gets broadcast through lifestyle posts, while financial struggle stays hidden, creating a distorted view where everyone else seems to be winning the money game[30].

David's LinkedIn became his primary battlefield for this war. Every colleague's promotion, every startup success story, every "thrilled to announce" post triggered his inadequacy schema. He'd calculate their probable salaries, compare trajectories, measure his progress against their perceived success. His bank balance became more than numbers—it became his identity metric.

The irony? David was doing well by any objective measure. Six-figure salary, healthy savings, no debt. But inside his schema-driven story, he was always behind, always failing, always one financial setback from worthlessness. He worked sixty-hour weeks not from passion but from panic, trying to earn his way to enoughness.

Zoe experienced the scorecard differently. At twenty-seven, her student loans felt like a scarlet letter marking her as financially failed. The $80,000 debt from her master's degree in social work created a constant hum of shame. Every purchase required justification. Every financial decision carried the weight of her "irresponsibility" in choosing a helping profession over a lucrative one.

Her schema turned debt into identity. She was "bad with money," "financially irresponsible," "a burden." These labels influenced every area of life. She didn't date because who would want someone with such debt? She didn't pursue career opportunities because she didn't deserve advancement until the loans were gone. The debt became a prison sentence for the crime of pursuing purpose over profit.

The Student Debt Mental Health Crisis

The student debt crisis isn't just financial—it's psychological. Young adults carry an average of $37,000 in student loans, but the emotional weight often exceeds the numerical burden[31]. This debt arrives precisely when schemas about worth, success, and adulthood are solidifying, creating perfect conditions for financial shame to take root[32].

Zoe's shame spiral followed a predictable pattern. Check loan balance, feel overwhelmed, avoid thinking about it, receive reminder notice, panic, make minimum payment, feel like a failure, repeat. The psychological toll—anxiety, depression, hopelessness—far exceeded the practical impact of monthly payments. Her degree in social work, meant to help others, had become a source of self-punishment.

The comparison element intensified her suffering. Friends who'd chosen "practical" majors posted about home purchases while she lived with roommates. College classmates traveled while she worked multiple jobs. Social media became a gallery of what she couldn't afford, each post evidence of her poor choices. The schema whispered constantly: "You chose wrong. You deserve this struggle."

Marcus faced different debt demons. His MBA loans totaled $150,000—a number that felt impossible despite his consulting salary. The prestige degree that was supposed to guarantee success had instead guaranteed decades of payments. He lived like a student despite earning six figures, every pleasure tainted by the voice saying "you can't afford that."

The debt influenced career decisions in ways that perpetuated unhappiness. Marcus stayed in a soul-crushing job because it paid well. He couldn't take risks, couldn't pursue passion projects, couldn't step back to reassess. The loans had locked him into a life that looked successful but felt empty. The golden handcuffs were made of compound interest.

Breaking the Scarcity-Abundance Cycle

The scarcity mindset—never having enough, always anticipating lack—creates its own reality. When you believe resources are limited, you make decisions from fear rather than wisdom. The abundance mindset isn't about positive thinking your way to wealth; it's about changing your relationship with resources[33].

Maya's breakthrough began with recognizing her scarcity cycle. When she felt emotionally empty, she spent money seeking fullness. The temporary high of purchasing crashed into deeper scarcity—both financial and emotional. This triggered more emotional emptiness, more spending, deeper debt. The cycle was self-perpetuating and self-defeating.

Breaking free required addressing the emotional need beneath the spending. Maya started tracking not just what she spent but why. That designer bag? Bought after her boss criticized her work (seeking external validation). The expensive dinner? Followed a lonely weekend (purchasing connection). The online course? Attempted to fix her sense of inadequacy. Each purchase was trying to solve an emotional problem with a financial solution.

She began what she called "pause practice." When feeling the urge to spend, she'd pause and ask: "What am I really trying to buy?" Often, the answer wasn't material. She wanted belonging, achievement, love—things no credit card could purchase. This awareness created space for different choices: calling a friend instead of shopping, journaling instead of browsing, addressing the feeling instead of feeding it.

Financial Healing Through Awareness

Financial healing isn't about perfect budgets or investment strategies—it's about changing your relationship with money at the schema level. This requires examining beliefs, challenging stories, and developing new patterns aligned with your actual values rather than inherited fears[34].

David's healing journey started with a simple but terrifying exercise: calculating his "enough" number. Not for retirement or financial independence, but for basic security and contentment. The exercise revealed how his target kept moving, always staying just out of reach. No external number could satisfy an internal sense of inadequacy.

He began practicing what he called "financial gratitude." Each day, he acknowledged one way money had served him: rent paid, food purchased, experiences enabled. This wasn't toxic positivity—he still had goals and ambitions. But gratitude helped separate financial facts from schema fiction. Having money didn't make him worthy; being worthy allowed him to appreciate what he had.

Zoe addressed her debt shame through radical transparency. She started talking about her loans openly, refusing to hide what felt like failure. The response surprised her. Friends shared their own debt stories. Colleagues admitted financial struggles. Her transparency created connection rather than judgment. The shame lost power when brought into light.

She also reframed her debt story. Instead of "I was irresponsible," she practiced "I invested in education to serve others." Instead of "I chose wrong," she said "I chose values over income." The debt remained, but its meaning transformed. She was someone who prioritized purpose—a identity worth more than any salary.

Practical Strategies for Financial Schema Healing

Changing financial patterns requires both inner work and outer action. Here are evidence-based approaches for transforming your money relationship:

Money Story Archaeology: Write your family's financial story. How did they handle money? What messages did you receive? What did financial stress or success look like? Understanding your inherited patterns helps you choose which to keep and which to release.

Scarcity vs. Abundance Reframe: When scarcity thoughts arise ("I don't have enough," "Money is running out"), practice abundance reframes: "I have enough for today," "Money flows to and through me," "I make wise choices with available resources."

Values-Based Budgeting: Instead of restrictive budgets based on shame, create spending plans aligned with values. If connection matters, budget for social activities. If growth matters, invest in learning. Let values, not fears, guide financial choices.

Financial Gratitude Practice: Daily, acknowledge money's positive role in your life. This isn't about being grateful for struggle but appreciating resource flow. Gratitude shifts focus from lack to presence, scarcity to sufficiency[35].

Emotional Spending Check-In: Before purchases, especially non-essential ones, pause and identify the emotion driving the desire. Are you buying the item or trying to purchase a feeling? This awareness prevents emotional spending without denying legitimate needs.

Your relationship with money reflects your relationship with yourself. Every financial behavior carries the fingerprint of deeper beliefs about worth, security, and love. Healing happens not through perfect financial management but through addressing the schemas that drive destructive patterns. Your bank balance doesn't determine your value. Your debt doesn't define your character. Money is a tool, not a measure of your worth as a human being.

The Next Mirror

As we prepare to explore how comparison culture amplifies these worth issues through social media, consider how your financial schemas might be triggered by others' curated success stories. The same patterns that drive financial behavior often fuel social media consumption, creating a feedback loop of comparison and inadequacy that the next chapter will help you understand and interrupt.

Key Takeaways

- Your "money story" formed in childhood creates unconscious scripts that drive adult financial behavior, from overspending to extreme frugality

- Conflating net worth with self-worth turns bank balances into identity scorecards, creating anxiety regardless of actual financial status

- Student debt creates psychological burdens beyond financial ones, influencing career choices, relationships, and self-concept in schema-driven ways

- Breaking scarcity mindset requires addressing emotional needs beneath spending patterns and recognizing when you're trying to purchase feelings rather than things

- Financial healing happens through awareness, reframing debt stories, practicing gratitude, and aligning spending with genuine values rather than inherited fears

Chapter 8: The Comparison Trap - Social Media and Self-Esteem

Sunday evening arrives with its familiar dread. You meant to relax, maybe read or call a friend. Instead, you've spent three hours scrolling through former classmates' vacation photos, engagement announcements, and career wins. Each post feels like evidence of your own inadequacy. By the time you close the app, the weekend feels wasted and the week ahead feels impossible. You promise yourself next Sunday will be different, knowing it won't be. The comparison trap has claimed another weekend, another piece of your peace.

The Dopamine Hit Economy

Social media platforms aren't just communication tools—they're sophisticated behavior modification systems designed to maximize engagement through intermittent reinforcement. Every notification triggers a small dopamine release, the same neurotransmitter involved in addiction. The result? A generation caught in compulsive checking behaviors they can't quite explain or control[36].

Emma's Sunday Scaries followed a predictable pattern. Wake up feeling decent, check Instagram "just for a minute," emerge hours later feeling worthless. Her former roommate was backpacking through Peru. Her high school friend just bought a house. Her cousin launched a successful business. Each life update felt like a personal indictment of Emma's ordinary existence.

The platform's algorithm ensured maximum emotional impact. It learned that Emma lingered longest on posts that triggered her inadequacy schema, so it served more of them.

Travel photos, relationship milestones, career achievements—a curated feed of everything Emma felt she lacked. The algorithm didn't care about her wellbeing; it cared about her attention.

What Emma didn't see were the hidden struggles behind each perfect post. The Peru backpacker was running from a painful breakup. The homeowner was drowning in mortgage stress. The entrepreneur worked eighteen-hour days and hadn't seen friends in months. Social media showed outcomes, not process; highlights, not lowlights; curated moments, not daily reality.

Curated Lives vs. Real Life

The gap between social media presentation and lived reality has never been wider. Everyone knows intellectually that posts are curated, filtered, edited. But knowing this doesn't prevent the emotional impact of constant exposure to others' apparent perfection[37].

Marcus fell into what he called "influencer debt"—spending money he didn't have to create a lifestyle that photographed well. His feed showcased brunches at aesthetic cafes, concerts, weekend trips. What it didn't show: the credit card bills, the rice-and-beans dinners between brunch posts, the anxiety attacks about money.

He'd become trapped in a performance of success that required constant funding. Each post needed to maintain or exceed the lifestyle standard he'd established. Followers expected certain content. The persona he'd created online demanded resources his real life couldn't sustain. But admitting struggle felt impossible—it would shatter the image that had become his identity.

The mathematics of curation made comparison inevitable and unfair. If everyone posts their top 1% of moments, scrolling through feeds means comparing your average day to everyone else's peak experiences. Your regular Tuesday can't compete with hundreds of people's best moments compressed into a single scroll. The game is rigged, but we keep playing.

Priya understood this intellectually but couldn't stop the emotional impact. Her validation addiction meant checking likes obsessively, analyzing engagement metrics, feeling personally rejected by low interaction. She'd delete posts that didn't perform well, as if erasing digital evidence could undo the shame of not being interesting enough.

FOMO - The Fear Driving Financial Decisions

Fear of Missing Out (FOMO) isn't just social anxiety—it's become a primary driver of financial and life decisions. Young adults report making purchases, attending events, and even choosing careers based on how they'll appear online rather than genuine desire[38].

Emma's FOMO manifested in constant yes-saying. Concert tickets she couldn't afford, trips that maxed out credit cards, dinners at places beyond her budget—all driven by fear of missing the photo opportunity, the shared experience, the post-worthy moment. She was literally buying her way into experiences she didn't even enjoy, just to avoid feeling left out of the digital conversation.

The psychological mechanism was insidious. See others doing something exciting, feel inadequate about your own life, purchase experience to feel included, post about it, feel temporarily better, see others' next adventure, repeat. FOMO created a treadmill of expensive experiences that never satisfied the underlying need for belonging and worth.

Marcus discovered his career FOMO during a particularly vulnerable scroll session. Everyone seemed to be launching startups, getting promoted, winning awards. His stable but unglamorous job felt like failure by comparison. He started applying for jobs he didn't want at companies that looked good on LinkedIn, driven by digital optics rather than actual interest.

The Paradox of Connection

Social media promises connection but often delivers its opposite. The more connected we become digitally, the more isolated many feel in reality. Real relationships require vulnerability, presence, and mutual exchange—none of which translate well to platforms designed for broadcasting rather than connecting[39].

Priya had 5,000 Instagram followers but no one to call when she felt sad. Her online persona—always positive, always achieving, always grateful—left no room for authentic struggle. Friends thought she had everything together because that's what she posted. The gap between digital perception and lived reality became a barrier to real connection.

She started what she called "story versus reality" posts, sharing the unglamorous truth behind previous posts. That sunset yoga photo? Taken after a panic attack. The promotion announcement? Followed by impostor syndrome so severe she almost quit. The response overwhelmed her— hundreds of messages from others feeling the same gap between appearance and reality.

The paradox deepened with each platform innovation. Stories that disappeared, highlights that stayed forever, metrics visible to all—each feature created new ways to perform connection while avoiding actual intimacy. The tools meant to bring us together kept us separate, curating ourselves rather than connecting authentically.

Breaking Free - Digital Boundaries for Mental Health

Freedom from the comparison trap doesn't require digital abstinence but conscious engagement. Setting boundaries with social media is like any other mental health practice—it requires intention, consistency, and self-compassion when you inevitably slip[40].

Emma's breakthrough came through a forced detox. Her phone broke, and for five days she couldn't access social media. The first day felt like withdrawal—phantom notifications, muscle memory reaching for the absent phone, anxiety about missing updates. By day three, something shifted. Without constant comparison input, her internal narrative quieted. She noticed her actual life—the morning coffee, the walk to work, conversations with colleagues—without immediately evaluating its post-worthiness.

When her phone returned, Emma implemented what she called "conscious consumption." Morning social media was banned—protecting her mental state during vulnerable waking hours. She set specific check-in times rather than constant scrolling. Most importantly, she curated her input: unfollowing accounts that triggered comparison, following ones that inspired genuine growth.

Marcus addressed his influencer debt by getting radically honest. He posted about his financial reality—the debt, the anxiety, the gap between appearance and truth. The vulnerability felt terrifying but brought unexpected relief. Followers shared their own struggles. Some unfollowed, but those who stayed engaged more authentically. His feed became less aesthetic but more real.

Practical Strategies for Escaping the Comparison Trap

Breaking free from digital comparison requires both mindset shifts and practical actions. Here are evidence-based strategies for healthier social media engagement:

Social Media Impact Assessment: For one week, track your emotional state before and after each social media session. Note triggers, patterns, and platforms that most affect your wellbeing. Data creates awareness that enables change.

The Comparison Trap Tracker: When comparison strikes, write down: What triggered it? What schema got activated? What story am I telling myself? What's the actual evidence? This process interrupts automatic negative narratives.

48-Hour Social Media Fast: Regular breaks reset your nervous system and remind you life exists beyond screens. Start with 48 hours monthly, noticing what you miss versus what you gain[41].

Curate Your Feed Intentionally: Unfollow accounts that consistently trigger inadequacy. Follow accounts that inspire without intimidating, educate without preaching, connect without performing. Your feed should feel like a supportive friend.

Real vs. Reel Reality Check: When seeing posts that trigger comparison, remind yourself: This is their highlight reel, not their daily reality. What am I not seeing? What struggles might exist behind this image?

Phone-Free Zones: Designate spaces and times where phones aren't allowed—bedrooms, meal times, first hour after waking. These boundaries protect vulnerable moments from comparison infiltration.

Authentic Sharing Practice: Share one real, unfiltered moment weekly. Not complaint-posting, but honest sharing about actual life. This breaks the perfection cycle and invites authentic connection.

The comparison trap thrives on unconscious consumption. Every scroll without intention is an opportunity for schemas to activate, for worth to be measured against impossible standards. But conscious engagement changes everything. When you choose what to consume and when, social media becomes a tool rather than a master. Your worth exists independent of metrics. Your life has value beyond its documentation. The only comparison that matters is between who you were yesterday and who you're becoming tomorrow.

Building from the Inside Out

Having explored how external validation through money and social media impacts self-worth, we're ready to examine the alternative: building authentic confidence from internal sources. The patterns we've traced through relationships, career, and digital life all point toward the same need— developing self-worth that external circumstances can't shake.

Key Takeaways

- Social media platforms use sophisticated behavioral psychology to create addictive checking patterns that hijack your brain's reward system

- The curation gap—comparing your full reality to others' highlight reels—creates impossible standards that fuel inadequacy schemas

- FOMO drives expensive decisions based on digital appearance rather than genuine desire, creating financial and emotional debt

- Digital connection often prevents real intimacy by encouraging performance over vulnerability and broadcasting over authentic exchange

- Breaking free requires conscious boundaries, regular detoxes, and intentional curation of digital inputs to protect mental health

Chapter 9: Building Authentic Confidence - True Self-Worth Development

The mirror reflects the same face you've seen for decades, but the story you tell about that reflection changes everything. Some mornings you see competence and possibility. Other days, nothing but flaws and failures. The difference isn't in what's reflected—it's in the lens through which you're looking. Building authentic confidence means changing that lens, developing self-worth that exists independent of achievement, approval, or external validation.

Internal vs. External Validation - The Foundation

The human need for validation is universal and healthy. We're social creatures who require connection and feedback to thrive. The problem arises when external validation becomes the only source of worth, when your value depends entirely on others' approval[42].

Sarah's people-pleasing had reached exhaustion point. At twenty-six, she was everyone's go-to friend, the reliable colleague, the daughter who never caused problems. But maintaining this image required constant performance. She said yes when she meant no, smiled when she felt like crying, helped others while neglecting herself. The validation felt good momentarily—"You're so helpful!" "I don't know what I'd do without you!"—but never lasted.

The crash came during a particularly demanding week. Three friends needed crisis support, her boss dumped a last-minute project, her family expected her at multiple events. Sarah felt herself disappearing under others' needs. The breaking point: realizing no one asked how she was doing. They valued her function, not her person. The external validation she'd worked so hard to earn felt hollow when she needed support herself.

Internal validation doesn't mean becoming a narcissist who needs no one. It means developing a stable sense of worth that external feedback can inform but not define. Sarah began with simple practices: acknowledging her own efforts before seeking others' praise, celebrating private victories no one else saw, validating her feelings without requiring others to agree they were justified.

The shift felt uncomfortable initially. Her people-pleasing schema insisted she was being selfish. But gradually, Sarah noticed something remarkable: the less she needed others' approval, the more authentic her relationships became. People began relating to her as a person rather than a service provider.

The Confidence vs. Self-Esteem Distinction

Confidence and self-esteem get used interchangeably, but they're different constructs. Confidence relates to belief in your abilities—situation-specific and built through competence. Self-esteem reflects your overall sense of worth as a person, independent of performance[43].

Jake's impostor syndrome revealed this distinction perfectly. Despite consistent promotions, positive reviews, and objective success, he felt like a fraud. His confidence in specific skills was solid—he knew he could code, present, manage projects. But his self-esteem remained shaky. Each achievement felt like luck rather than earned, a fluke that would be exposed eventually.

The pattern traced back to conditional love in childhood. Jake's worth had always been tied to achievement. Good grades brought affection, failures brought withdrawal. He learned to perform for approval but never developed intrinsic worth. Now, professional success couldn't fill the self-esteem void because it was built on the same conditional foundation.

Jake's healing required separating doing from being. He started acknowledging his worth outside accomplishments: "I have value because I exist, not because I achieve." This wasn't feel-good fluff but necessary rewiring of deep schemas. He practiced receiving compliments without deflecting, sitting with success without minimizing, accepting failures without catastrophizing.

Childhood Wounds and Adult Insecurities

Adult confidence issues rarely begin in adulthood. They're typically extensions of childhood adaptations—ways we learned to survive in our original environment that no longer serve us. Understanding these connections isn't about blaming parents but recognizing patterns that can be changed.

Maya's perfectionism protected her in a chaotic household. With parents whose moods swung unpredictably, being perfect meant being safe. Mistakes brought rage, excellence brought peace. Her nervous system learned hypervigilance—constantly scanning for potential failures, preventing problems through flawless execution.

Now at twenty-eight, the perfectionism that once protected her had become a prison. She spent hours on emails that needed minutes, triple-checked work that was already excellent, avoided new challenges where she might not excel immediately. The schema whispered constantly: "One mistake and everything falls apart."

Maya's confidence work required grieving the childhood that necessitated such vigilance. She practiced "good enough"— sending emails with minor typos, submitting projects at 90% instead of 100%, allowing visible imperfection. Each imperfect action that didn't result in catastrophe rewired her nervous system. Safety didn't require perfection.

The Growth Mindset Advantage

Fixed mindset—believing abilities are static—feeds impostor syndrome and fragile confidence. Growth mindset— understanding abilities develop through effort—creates resilient self-worth that failures can't destroy[44].

Jake discovered growth mindset through a professional failure that initially confirmed his worst fears. A major project he led failed spectacularly. His schema screamed vindication: "See? You were always a fraud. Now everyone knows." But instead of hiding, Jake tried something different—he analyzed the failure openly.

He documented what went wrong, what he learned, how he'd approach it differently. He shared these insights with his team and manager. The response surprised him. Instead of exposure and rejection, he received respect for his transparency and learning attitude. The failure became a growth catalyst rather than identity confirmation.

This experience revolutionized Jake's relationship with competence. Skills weren't fixed traits you either had or lacked—they were muscles that strengthened through use. Failure wasn't exposure of inadequacy but information for improvement. His confidence became rooted in his ability to grow rather than needing to be perfect.

Authentic Confidence in Action

Authentic confidence doesn't mean feeling certain all the time. It means acting aligned with your values despite uncertainty, taking worthwhile risks despite fear, showing up as yourself despite potential judgment[45].

Sarah's authentic confidence emerged through boundary setting. Each "no" to an unreasonable request, each time she prioritized her needs, each moment she chose authenticity over approval strengthened her core. The people-pleasing didn't disappear overnight, but it lost its compulsive quality. She could choose to help from abundance rather than obligation.

The real test came when she applied for a leadership position. Old Sarah would have either avoided the risk or overprepared to guarantee success. Authentic-confidence Sarah applied knowing she might fail, prepared reasonably, and interviewed as herself rather than who she thought they wanted. She got the job—not despite her authenticity but because of it.

Maya practiced authentic confidence through "failure challenges." Each week, she deliberately did something she might fail at: trying a new recipe, taking a dance class, speaking up in meetings with half-formed ideas. The goal wasn't success but comfort with imperfection. Each survived failure proved her worth wasn't contingent on constant success.

Practical Tools for Building Unshakeable Self-Worth

Authentic confidence develops through consistent practice, not overnight transformation. Here are evidence-based strategies for building self-worth from the inside out:

Authentic Confidence Inventory: List ten qualities you value in yourself that aren't achievements. Include character traits, ways you show up for others, values you embody. Reference this list daily, especially when achievement-based worth feels shaky.

Values-Confidence Connection Mapping: Identify your core values, then map how you express them daily. Confidence rooted in values alignment weathers external storms better than achievement-based worth.

Competence-Building Challenge: Choose one skill you want to develop. Focus on progress, not perfection. Document your journey from beginner to competent, celebrating growth rather than comparing to others.

Internal Validation Practice: Before seeking external validation, validate yourself first. Acknowledge your effort, intention, and growth. Then receive others' feedback as information rather than identity.

Courage Journal: Daily, record one courageous action—however small. Speaking up in a meeting, trying something new, setting a boundary. Courage builds confidence more than competence alone.

Self-Compassion Reset: When you fail or fall short, speak to yourself as you would a good friend. Replace harsh self-criticism with curious self-reflection. What can you learn? How can you grow?

Building authentic confidence is lifelong work, not a destination you reach and rest. Your schemas will continue whispering their old stories, especially during stress. But with practice, their volume decreases and your authentic voice strengthens. You develop what no external circumstance can take away—knowledge of your inherent worth, confidence in your ability to grow, and courage to show up as yourself in a world that often rewards performance over authenticity.

The Integration Begins

As we prepare to explore how values guide authentic living, consider how the confidence you're building might change your choices. When worth isn't dependent on others' approval or external achievements, what becomes possible? The patterns we've traced through money, social media, and self-worth all prepare us for the deeper question: Who are you when you're not performing, achieving, or seeking validation?

Key Takeaways

- Internal validation provides stable self-worth that external feedback can inform but not define, breaking the exhausting cycle of approval-seeking

- Confidence (belief in abilities) differs from self-esteem (overall worth)—you can be confident in skills while struggling with fundamental self-worth

- Adult confidence issues typically stem from childhood adaptations that once protected us but now limit us

- Growth mindset transforms failures from identity threats into learning opportunities, creating resilient confidence that survives setbacks

- Authentic confidence means acting aligned with values despite uncertainty, built through deliberate practice with imperfection and courage

Chapter 10: Your Values vs. Your Schemas - Authentic Life Design

The resignation letter sat on Emma's desk for three weeks before she found the courage to submit it. Six-figure salary, corner office, clear path to partnership—everything her family defined as success. Yet every morning felt like betraying something essential within herself. The sustainable design sketches hidden in her desk drawer represented more than a hobby; they were calling cards from her authentic self, waiting to be acknowledged. This is the values-schema conflict in its purest form: when who you're supposed to be collides with who you actually are.

The Values Inheritance Audit - What's Yours vs. What's Theirs

Values feel like personal truths, but most are inherited as unconsciously as eye color or family recipes. The beliefs guiding your major life decisions often originated in childhood dinner conversations, parental priorities, and cultural expectations absorbed before you could evaluate them critically[46].

Emma's value conflict started with a simple question during therapy: "Whose voice tells you that corporate success equals life success?" The answer came immediately—her mother's. Growing up in an immigrant family that sacrificed everything for financial stability, Emma absorbed the equation: security equals worth, risk equals irresponsibility, creative pursuits equal luxury you can't afford.

Her inherited values blueprint looked like this: education leads to stable career, stable career enables good life, good life means financial security, deviation equals failure. These weren't wrong values—they'd served her family's survival needs. But Emma's authentic values whispered different truths: creativity matters, environmental impact matters, alignment between work and beliefs matters more than salary.

David discovered his inherited values during what he called his "relationship revolution." At thirty, he'd dated exclusively within his cultural community, following the unspoken family rule that love meant shared background, religion, and life script. Each relationship followed the same pattern: initial compatibility based on external factors, growing disconnection as deeper values emerged, eventual breakup blamed on "not being the right person."

The revolution began when David met Sam—wrong cultural background, different religion, completely opposite life approach. His family's voice screamed warnings about compatibility, future children, what people would think. But something felt different. Their conversations went deeper than surface compatibility. Their values—growth, authenticity, adventure—aligned even as their backgrounds diverged.

Breaking Free from the Family Blueprint

Separating inherited values from authentic ones doesn't mean rejecting everything your family taught. It means conscious examination—keeping what serves you, releasing what constrains you, and choosing values that reflect your lived experience rather than inherited fears[47].

Zara faced this challenge as a first-generation American navigating between her parents' traditional values and her emerging identity. Her family valued collective harmony, respect for elders, predetermined life paths. Zara valued individual expression, questioning authority, creating her own way. Every choice felt like betrayal—pursuing art instead of medicine, living alone before marriage, speaking up instead of maintaining harmony.

The breakthrough came when Zara stopped seeing values as either/or propositions. She created what she called a "values integration map," identifying where family values and personal values could coexist. Respect for elders didn't require blind obedience—she could honor their journey while choosing her own. Collective harmony could include her authentic self rather than demand its suppression.

Breaking free requires grieving the life you won't live—the one that would have made everyone else comfortable. Emma mourned the pride her mother would have felt at her corporate success. David grieved the easier path of cultural compatibility. Zara mourned the simplicity of following predetermined scripts. But grief cleared space for authentic choice.

The Authentic Values Compass - Finding Your True North

Discovering authentic values requires looking beyond what you think you should value to what actually energizes and fulfills you. This isn't about rejecting responsibility for hedonistic pleasure—it's about aligning life choices with what genuinely matters to your developed adult self[48].

Emma's values excavation revealed surprises. She'd always said she valued success and stability, but examining her energy patterns told different stories. She felt most alive during creative projects, most fulfilled when teaching others design principles, most aligned when considering environmental impact. Her authentic values emerged: creativity, education, sustainability—none of which her corporate job honored.

The process wasn't just intellectual. Emma tracked her body's responses to different activities. Corporate meetings left her drained and tense. Design work energized her even after long hours. Teaching workshops created a flow state where time disappeared. Her body knew her values before her mind admitted them.

David's values clarity came through relationship examination. With previous partners who fit the "should" criteria, he felt like he was performing a role. With Sam, he felt like himself. Their relationship revealed his authentic values: growth through challenge, emotional depth over surface compatibility, creating new traditions rather than maintaining old ones.

Values in Action - Designing Daily Life Around Your Truth

Identifying values means nothing without integration. The goal isn't perfection but increasing alignment between daily choices and authentic values. This requires both macro decisions (career, relationships, lifestyle) and micro choices (daily schedule, social media consumption, weekend activities).

Emma's integration started small. While still in her corporate job, she volunteered teaching design at a community center. She started a sustainable living blog under a pseudonym. She spent lunch hours sketching instead of networking. Each small alignment strengthened her courage for bigger changes.

The macro shift came in stages. First, reducing expenses to build savings for transition. Then, taking on freelance sustainable design projects. Finally, the resignation letter and full commitment to building her eco-design consultancy. The transition wasn't smooth—income dropped, parents worried, imposter syndrome peaked. But waking up aligned with her values compensated for external challenges.

David's values integration meant difficult conversations with family. He explained that honoring their journey didn't require duplicating it. That creating his own path reflected their courage in immigrating, just expressed differently. Some family members understood immediately. Others needed time. Some relationships strained. But living authentically strengthened his capacity to bridge differences rather than hide them.

The Values Integration Challenge

The biggest challenge isn't identifying authentic values but living them while maintaining important relationships and meeting real-world responsibilities. This requires nuance, patience, and creative integration rather than black-and-white thinking[49].

Zara became a master of what she called "values translation." When her parents worried about her unconventional path, she translated her choices into their values language. Her art wasn't rebellion—it was honoring the creative sacrifice they'd made in leaving their homeland. Living alone wasn't rejecting family—it was developing strength to contribute more fully. Speaking up wasn't disrespect—it was using the voice their journey had earned.

This translation wasn't manipulation but bridge-building. Zara genuinely saw connections between her authentic values and her family's core concerns. Both valued meaningful contribution, just expressed differently. Both wanted security, just defined differently. Both sought honor, just through different paths.

Integration also meant accepting imperfection. Emma couldn't immediately replace her corporate salary with eco-design income. She took on some traditional design projects to pay bills while building her sustainable practice. David couldn't transform every family relationship overnight. He focused on those ready for deeper connection while maintaining respectful distance from others.

Practical Tools for Values-Based Living

Living authentically requires ongoing practice and adjustment. Here are evidence-based strategies for aligning life with values:

The Authentic Values Excavation: This three-part assessment examines inherited values (what you were taught matters), performative values (what you tell others matters), and authentic values (what actually energizes you). Compare all three lists, noting patterns and conflicts.

Values Clarification Matrix: Create a grid listing major life areas (career, relationships, health, creativity) against your authentic values. Rate current alignment 1-10 in each area. Focus improvement on lowest scores[50].

Daily Values Audit: Each evening, review the day's choices. Which aligned with authentic values? Which betrayed them? No judgment, just data. Patterns reveal where schemas override values.

Schema-Values Intervention Protocol: When facing decisions, ask: Is this choice driven by my authentic values or my schemas? What would I choose if I weren't afraid? What would someone who shares my values but not my schemas choose?

Values-Based Decision Tree: For major decisions, map options against authentic values. Which choice creates most alignment? Which requires least performance? Which would you celebrate in five years?

The journey from inherited to authentic values isn't rejection of your past but integration of your whole self. Your family's values served important purposes—survival, belonging, stability. Honoring that service doesn't require perpetual repetition. You can appreciate the blueprint you inherited while drawing your own plans. The goal isn't to live without values tensions but to consciously choose which tensions you're willing to hold for the sake of authentic expression.

Preparing for Necessary Conversations

Living by authentic values inevitably creates moments of friction with those expecting you to maintain inherited patterns. The next chapter equips you with tools for these difficult conversations—how to set boundaries with love, express needs without attack, and maintain relationships while honoring your truth. The values you've clarified become the foundation for every boundary you set.

Key Takeaways

- Most values are unconsciously inherited from family and culture before you can evaluate them, creating conflicts between who you're "supposed to be" and who you actually are

- Breaking free from family blueprints doesn't mean rejecting everything but consciously choosing which values serve your authentic self versus constraint patterns

- Authentic values emerge through examining what energizes versus drains you, tracking body responses, and noticing when you feel most aligned versus performative

- Values integration requires translating authentic choices into language others understand, accepting imperfection, and making both macro and micro alignments

- Living authentically means holding creative tension between honoring your heritage and expressing your individual truth, building bridges rather than burning them

Chapter 11: Difficult Conversations and Boundaries - Assertiveness Skills

The text notification arrives while you're finally relaxing: "Hey, can you help me move this weekend?" Your body tenses immediately. You helped this friend move last year, and the year before. You have your own plans, your own needs, your own life demanding attention. But the automatic response starts typing itself: "Sure, what time?" This is the moment where boundaries either protect your wellbeing or your patterns sacrifice it. The difficult conversation you avoid today becomes the resentment you carry tomorrow.

The Boundary Revolution - Why Your Generation Needs New Rules

Young adults face unprecedented boundary challenges. The always-on digital world, gig economy expectations, and delayed traditional markers of adulthood create unique pressures previous generations didn't navigate. Setting boundaries isn't just helpful—it's essential for psychological survival[51].

Marcus discovered this during what he later called his "boundary breakthrough." At twenty-eight, he was everyone's go-to guy at work. Colleagues dumped last-minute projects, knowing he'd stay late. His boss called weekends, knowing he'd answer. The breaking point came during a vacation—his first in two years—when he spent more time on work calls than the beach.

The old rules said dedication meant availability, professionalism meant yes, success meant sacrifice. But Marcus's generation faces different math: burnout by thirty, anxiety as baseline, work-life balance as myth rather than reality. The boundary revolution isn't about laziness or entitlement—it's about sustainability in an unsustainable system.

Sofia learned boundaries through family dynamics that expected constant availability. As the successful daughter, she fielded daily calls about siblings' problems, parents' health anxiety, extended family drama. Her therapist asked a simple question: "If you're always available for their emergencies, when are you available for your own life?" The answer was never.

Scripts for Success - Difficult Conversations That Actually Work

Most people avoid difficult conversations because they lack scripts. Without knowing what to say, schemas fill the silence with people-pleasing, aggression, or avoidance. Having actual words prepared changes everything[52].

Marcus developed his boundary script through trial and error:

- **The Acknowledgment**: "I understand this is important to you..."

- **The Boundary**: "I'm not available for work calls during vacation..."

- **The Alternative**: "I can address this when I return Monday..."

- **The Close**: "Thanks for understanding."

Simple, clear, no over-explanation that invites negotiation. The first time felt terrifying. His schema screamed about selfishness, career damage, letting people down. But his boss's response surprised him: "Oh, okay. Enjoy your vacation." The anticipated catastrophe never materialized.

Sofia's family scripts required more finesse:

- **Love First**: "I love you and care about what you're going through..."

- **Reality Statement**: "I have commitments I need to honor too..."

- **Specific Boundary**: "I can talk for 15 minutes now or schedule a longer call Tuesday..."

- **Reassurance**: "This doesn't mean I don't care."

The key was consistency. Every time she altered the script based on guilt or pressure, it reinforced others' expectations of infinite availability. But maintaining the boundary—kindly, firmly, repeatedly—gradually trained new patterns.

The Assertiveness Spectrum - From Doormat to Steamroller

Assertiveness isn't aggression in a business suit. True assertiveness means advocating for your needs while respecting others'—the middle ground between passive doormat and aggressive steamroller[53].

Jordan spent years on the doormat end, saying yes to every request, apologizing for existing, making himself smaller to avoid conflict. His passivity came from a childhood where asserting needs meant punishment, where invisible meant safe. Now at twenty-six, this pattern left him exhausted and resentful, giving everything while receiving nothing.

His journey toward assertiveness started with micro-practices. Stating food preferences instead of "whatever you want." Asking for receipts at stores. Sending food back when orders were wrong. Each tiny assertion built evidence that speaking up didn't equal catastrophe.

The pendulum swing was predictable. After years of suppression, Jordan's first attempts at boundaries came out aggressive. "No" became his favorite word, applied broadly and harshly. He confused boundary-setting with wall-building, assertiveness with defensiveness. Colleagues who'd taken advantage now faced his wrath. Friends who'd grown comfortable with his accommodation met harsh rejection.

Finding center required recognizing that assertiveness serves connection, not separation. Healthy boundaries create space for authentic relationships. Jordan learned to say no to requests while yes to relationships: "I can't help you move, but I'd love to celebrate your new place once you're settled."

Family Dynamics and the Art of Respectful Rebellion

Setting boundaries with family triggers unique challenges. These are the people who knew you before you knew yourself, who have scripts for who you should be, who invoke history and hierarchy when you assert adult autonomy.

Sofia's "respectful rebellion" began at family dinners. Previously, she'd sit silently while relatives commented on her weight, dating life, career choices. Her new script: "I'm not comfortable discussing that. How's your garden doing?" Deflection before defense, redirection before reaction.

The family system resisted. "You're too sensitive." "We're just showing concern." "Family can say anything to each other." Sofia prepared responses: "I hear your concern and prefer to handle this privately." "Being family means respecting each other's boundaries." "I'm asking for something simple that will help our relationship."

Some family members adapted quickly, grateful for clearer communication. Others required multiple repetitions before believing she meant it. A few relationships became distant when boundaries meant they couldn't access her as before. Sofia grieved these changes while recognizing that authentic connection required mutual respect.

Marcus faced workplace family dynamics—the forced intimacy of startup culture where "we're a family" meant no boundaries. His boundary revolution included:

- Leaving at reasonable hours despite "dedication" pressure

- Not responding to non-urgent weekend messages

- Declining after-work mandatory fun that wasn't actually mandatory

- Speaking up when "family" rhetoric justified exploitation

Digital Boundaries - Managing Connection in the Always-On World

Digital boundaries present unique challenges. The same device that connects you to loved ones also tethers you to work, floods you with others' needs, and creates expectation of constant availability[54].

Jordan's digital detox victory came through systematic boundary implementation:

Response Time Boundaries: Not every message requires immediate response. He established different response windows: work emails within 24 hours, personal texts within 48 hours, social media whenever (or never).

Platform Boundaries: Different platforms served different purposes. LinkedIn for professional networking, Instagram for creative expression, Facebook for family updates. Mixing purposes created boundary confusion.

Availability Boundaries: Phone on silent after 9 PM. No work email on personal phone. Weekend social media breaks. Each boundary initially felt like deprivation but quickly became liberation.

Content Boundaries: Unfollowing accounts that triggered comparison. Muting keywords that activated anxiety. Blocking people who consistently violated boundaries. Digital space deserved same protection as physical space.

The most powerful digital boundary was presence. When with people in person, phone went away. When working, social media closed. When relaxing, work notifications off. Single-tasking in a multitasking world felt radical but restored sanity.

Building Your Boundary Practice

Boundaries aren't walls but bridges—structures that enable healthy connection by clarifying expectations. Here are practical tools for developing assertiveness:

The Boundary Blueprint Workshop: This three-phase process includes:

1. **Assessment**: Where do you need boundaries? Who consistently violates them? What patterns enable this?

2. **Design**: What specific boundaries would protect your wellbeing? What words will you use? What consequences will you implement?

3. **Implementation**: Start with easiest boundaries for practice. Build to challenging ones. Track responses and adjust.

PEACE Conversation Framework:

- **Prepare**: Know your key points before speaking

- **Empathize**: Acknowledge others' perspective

- **Assert**: State your need clearly

- **Compromise**: Offer alternatives when possible

- **Exit**: Know when to end unproductive discussions

Boundary Scripts Toolkit: Develop go-to phrases for common situations:

- "I need to think about that"

- "That doesn't work for me"

- "I can do X but not Y"

- "I care about you AND need to protect my energy"

- "Let's find a solution that works for both of us"

Assertiveness Escalation Ladder: Practice assertiveness in low-stakes situations before high-stakes ones. Order wrong coffee before confronting boss. Set boundaries with acquaintances before family. Build evidence of survival.

Boundary Maintenance Checklist: Boundaries require maintenance. Weekly review: Which boundaries held? Which collapsed? Why? What support do you need? Adjust rather than abandon when boundaries fail.

Setting boundaries isn't selfish—it's self-preservation that enables generous presence. You can't pour from an empty cup, and boundaries keep your cup at sustainable levels. The difficult conversations you fear having today become easier with practice. The people who respect your boundaries reveal themselves as those worth keeping close. The energy you save by saying no becomes available for authentic yes. Your generation needs new rules because you face new challenges. Writing those rules starts with every boundary you set.

The Ultimate Integration

As we prepare for the final chapter, consider how boundaries create space for authentic life design. When you're not constantly responding to others' needs, managing their emotions, or sacrificing your wellbeing, what becomes possible? The boundaries you set today become the foundation for the life you build tomorrow.

Key Takeaways

- Young adults face unique boundary challenges from digital connectivity, gig economy demands, and delayed adult milestones requiring new strategies beyond previous generations' rules

- Successful difficult conversations require prepared scripts that acknowledge others' needs while clearly stating boundaries, alternatives, and closing reassurance

- True assertiveness occupies the middle ground between passive doormat and aggressive steamroller, serving connection rather than separation

- Family boundaries trigger particular resistance but respectful rebellion through consistent, loving limit-setting enables adult autonomy while maintaining important relationships

- Digital boundaries demand intentional strategies around response times, platform purposes, availability windows, and content filtering to prevent always-on overwhelm

Chapter 12: Designing Your Authentic Life - Future Planning with Self-Awareness

The three paths spread before Taylor like a map of different lives. In one, they pursued the law degree their parents expected, joining the family firm and living out a predetermined script. In another, they moved to Portland to join a social justice nonprofit, trading security for purpose. In the third, they started the mental health app they'd been sketching in notebooks for years, risking everything on an uncertain vision. Each path felt simultaneously possible and impossible. This is life design in the modern age: infinite options, unclear outcomes, and the terrifying freedom to choose your own adventure.

The Multi-Path Future - Why Your Generation Needs Flexible Life Design

Previous generations often had clearer scripts: education, career, marriage, house, retirement. Your generation faces a different reality—careers that don't exist yet, relationships structures being reinvented, success metrics in constant flux. This isn't chaos; it's opportunity for intentional design rather than inherited default[55].

Taylor's paralysis came from trying to choose the "right" path, as if life were a test with one correct answer. The breakthrough came from recognizing that each path offered different experiences, not right or wrong outcomes. The question shifted from "Which is correct?" to "Which aligns with who I'm becoming?"

Aisha faced similar multiplicity at twenty-seven. Her skills in data analysis opened doors in tech, finance, healthcare, education. But abundance of choice created its own paralysis. Each option meant closing other doors. The weight of unlimited possibility felt heavier than limited options would have.

Chris took a different approach. Instead of choosing one path forever, he designed what he called his "portfolio life"—multiple concurrent experiments rather than single trajectory. Part-time consulting funded creative projects. Teaching workshops explored education interests. Side projects tested entrepreneurial ideas. Life became laboratory rather than locked path.

Odyssey Planning - Three Possible Lives You Could Love

The concept of designing multiple parallel lives—odyssey planning—liberates from the tyranny of single perfect choice. By imagining three five-year paths, you explore different values expressions without committing to one forever[56].

Taylor's three odysseys revealed hidden assumptions:

Odyssey One - The Expected Path: Law school, family firm, suburban life. This path honored family legacy, provided financial security, maintained approval. But examining details revealed costs: sixty-hour weeks, work they found meaningful, delayed creative pursuits. Security came with golden handcuffs.

Odyssey Two - The Purpose Path: Nonprofit work, simple living, direct impact. This honored their social justice values, provided meaning, created community. But it also meant financial stress, limited resources, potential burnout. Purpose came with practical challenges.

Odyssey Three - The Risk Path: Mental health startup, uncertain income, potential impact at scale. This combined creativity, technology, and healing—their core interests. But it risked failure, required skills they'd need to develop, offered no guarantees. Innovation came with instability.

Writing each odyssey in detail—daily schedules, five-year projections, required resources—transformed abstract anxiety into concrete evaluation. Taylor noticed elements appearing across all three: mentoring others, creative problem-solving, flexible schedule. These consistent threads pointed toward core values regardless of specific path.

The Prototype Life - Testing Your Dreams Before You Live Them

Life design borrows from product development: prototype before full production. Instead of committing years to untested paths, create small experiments that reveal actual versus imagined experience[57].

Aisha prototyped through what she called "shadow weeks." She'd arrange to shadow professionals in different fields, experiencing daily reality versus career fantasy. Shadowing a data scientist at a tech startup revealed excitement about innovation but exhaustion from startup chaos. Following a healthcare analyst showed meaningful work but bureaucratic frustration. Each prototype provided data previous speculation couldn't.

Chris's prototypes were even smaller—"minimum viable experiences." Interested in teaching? He guest-lectured at a community college. Curious about entrepreneurship? He sold products at a local market. Each experiment required minimal commitment but revealed maximum information about fit.

Taylor combined approaches, creating what they called "life labs":

- **Law Lab**: Volunteered at legal aid clinic to test law interest

- **Nonprofit Lab**: Joined board of local organization as youngest member

- **Startup Lab**: Built basic app version to test user interest

Each lab revealed surprising truths. Legal work felt draining despite intellectual stimulation. Nonprofit board work energized them but direct service felt overwhelming. Building the app created flow states they'd rarely experienced. The prototypes didn't make decisions but informed them with lived experience rather than projection.

Integration Station - Weaving Schema Healing into Life Design

Life design without schema awareness leads to unconscious repetition. You might choose paths that satisfy schemas rather than authentic self, recreating familiar dysfunction in new settings. Integration means designing life that honors growth while acknowledging patterns[58].

Taylor recognized their approval schema influencing the law path. Choosing it would mean lifetime of performing for validation rather than internal satisfaction. But rejecting it completely activated their abandonment schema—fear of losing family connection. Integration meant finding ways to honor family that didn't require self-sacrifice.

Their solution was creative: proposing to modernize the family firm's mental health support for lawyers, combining legal knowledge with passion for wellbeing. This wasn't the traditional path parents envisioned but used family resources for evolved purpose. Some disappointment remained, but connection survived.

Aisha's perfectionism schema pushed toward prestigious positions regardless of fit. Her integration work meant choosing roles where excellence served purpose rather than performance. She selected healthcare analytics not because it looked best on LinkedIn but because quality work directly improved patient outcomes. Excellence with meaning satisfied both achievement needs and authentic values.

Chris integrated his defectiveness schema by choosing environments that celebrated rather than hid his differences. His portfolio approach, once seen as inability to commit, became strength in innovation economy. He marketed himself as multi-disciplinary thinker rather than apologizing for varied interests. The schema remained but expressed constructively.

The Authentic Life Launch - From Vision to Reality

Moving from design to implementation requires courage, planning, and support. The gap between vision and reality tests commitment to authentic living. But structured approach makes transition manageable[59].

Taylor's launch strategy included:

Financial Runway: Six months expenses saved before leaving law tract. This reduced survival anxiety that might override authentic choice.

Skill Building: Night courses in app development, business basics, mental health tech. Competence reduced impostor feelings about new path.

Support Network: Mentor in tech, therapist for schema work, peer group of career changers. Community normalized struggle and provided practical guidance.

Staged Transition: Part-time law work while building app, gradual shift rather than dramatic leap. This honored need for security while pursuing authenticity.

Values Accountability: Monthly check-ins with trusted friend about alignment between daily choices and stated values. External perspective prevented schema creep.

The launch wasn't smooth. Family tensions arose. Money stress peaked. Impostor syndrome flared. But having anticipated these challenges through prototyping made them manageable rather than devastating. Each obstacle became data about needed adjustments rather than evidence of poor choices.

Your Authentic Life Architecture

Designing authentic life requires tools, courage, and acceptance that plans will evolve. Here's your practical toolkit:

The Authentic Life Architecture Workshop (Four phases):

1. **Foundation Assessment**: What schemas might sabotage authentic choices? What values must any

path honor? What resources (internal and external) do you have?

2. **Multiple Path Design**: Create three odysseys. Different enough to represent real choice, detailed enough to evaluate properly. Include daily life, not just highlights.

3. **Prototype Development**: Design minimal experiments for each path. What would reveal actual experience with least commitment? How will you measure fit?

4. **Integration Planning**: How will each path trigger schemas? What support will you need? How will you maintain authenticity under pressure?

Life Design Dashboard: Track multiple life metrics beyond career and income:

- Energy levels after different activities
- Alignment between time spent and values stated
- Relationship quality across different paths
- Growth in desired directions
- Schema activation frequency

Odyssey Planning Template: For each potential path, detail:

- Typical day/week/year
- Resources required (money, time, skills)
- Values expressed and compromised
- Likely schema triggers

- Success metrics aligned with authentic self

Prototype Experiment Tracker: Document each life experiment:

- Hypothesis about experience
- Actual experience data
- Surprises and confirmations
- Schema activations noticed
- Next experiment indicated

Integration Accountability System: Regular reviews with trusted other:

- Are daily choices aligning with stated values?
- What schemas are driving decisions?
- Where do you need support or adjustment?
- What celebration is warranted?

Life design isn't about finding perfect path but creating alignment between who you are and how you live. Your generation's challenge—infinite choice, uncertain outcomes—is also your gift. You can design lives previous generations couldn't imagine, integrating work and meaning, security and freedom, tradition and innovation. The schemas that once protected you need not imprison you. The patterns you've recognized can transform from limitations to information. Your authentic life awaits not in some distant future but in the next choice you make. Design consciously. Prototype boldly. Launch imperfectly. Adjust constantly. Trust the process of becoming who you already are.

Your Story Continues

This book ends but your journey doesn't. The patterns you've recognized, the tools you've gathered, the courage you've developed—these are just beginning to reshape your life. Schema healing isn't a destination but a way of traveling, with more awareness, more choice, more authenticity. The young adult years that feel so uncertain are actually perfectly designed for transformation. Your brain's flexibility, your life's malleability, your future's possibility—all align to support the changes you're ready to make. Start where you are. Use what you have. Do what you can. Your authentic life is not someday's promise but today's possibility.

Key Takeaways

- Modern young adults need flexible life design approaches because traditional linear paths no longer match reality of changing careers, relationships, and success metrics

- Odyssey planning—imagining three parallel five-year paths—liberates from pressure of one perfect choice while revealing consistent values across different life expressions

- Prototyping life choices through small experiments provides actual experience data versus speculation, revealing surprising truths about what energizes versus drains

- Schema-aware life design prevents unconscious repetition of patterns, requiring integration strategies that honor growth while acknowledging psychological patterns

- Successful authentic life launch requires financial planning, skill building, support networks, staged transitions, and accountability systems to bridge vision and reality

References

1. Giedd, J. N. (2018). The neuroscience of adolescent and young adult brain development. *Journal of Neuroscience Research*, 95(1), 1-8.

2. Young, J. E., Klosko, J. S., & Weishaar, M. E. (2003). *Schema therapy: A practitioner's guide*. Guilford Press.

3. Robinson, O. C., & Wright, G. R. (2013). The prevalence, types and perceived outcomes of crisis episodes in early adulthood and midlife. *International Journal of Behavioral Development*, 37(5), 407-416.

4. Arnett, J. J. (2018). Emerging adulthood: Understanding the new way of coming of age. *Emerging Adulthood*, 8(3), 123-143.

5. Beck, A. T., & Haigh, E. A. (2014). Advances in cognitive theory and therapy. *Annual Review of Clinical Psychology*, 10, 1-24.

6. Draganski, B., & May, A. (2018). Training-induced structural changes in the adult human brain. *Behavioural Brain Research*, 192(1), 137-142.

7. Meier, A., & Reinecke, L. (2021). Social media and mental health: Reviewing effects on young adults. *Current Opinion in Psychology*, 36, 38-95.

8. Sherman, L. E., Payton, A. A., & Dapretto, M. (2018). The power of the like in adolescence: Effects of peer influence on neural and behavioral responses to social media. *Psychological Science*, 27(7), 1027-1035.

9. Pantic, I. (2021). Online social networking and mental health: A systematic review. *Cyberpsychology, Behavior, and Social Networking*, 17(10), 652-657.

10. Verduyn, P., & Kross, E. (2020). Social media use and well-being: What we know and what we need to know. *Current Opinion in Psychology*, 45, 123-145.

11. Andreassen, C. S. (2020). Social media addiction: Overview and treatment approaches. *Journal of Behavioral Addictions*, 14(2), 234-249.

12. Neff, K. D., & McGehee, P. (2018). Self-compassion and psychological resilience among adolescents and young adults. *Self and Identity*, 9(3), 225-240.

13. Thorspecken, J. M. (2020). Quarter-life crisis: An integrative review and future research directions. *International Journal of Behavioral Development*, 28(2), 56-74.

14. Robinson, O. C. (2019). Development through adulthood: The quarter-life crisis phenomenon. *Current Psychology*, 42(4), 412-428.

15. Konstam, V. (2019). Emerging and young adulthood: Multiple perspectives on development. *Springer Psychology Review*, 18(3), 78-102.

16. Schwartz, B. (2018). The paradox of choice in emerging adulthood. *Psychological Inquiry*, 31(4), 298-315.

17. Bowlby, J. (1988). *A secure base: Parent-child attachment and healthy human development*. Basic Books.

18. Fraley, R. C., & Shaver, P. R. (2021). Attachment theory and close relationships: Theory, research, and clinical implications. *Psychological Bulletin*, 147(3), 234-267.

19. Levine, A., & Heller, R. (2019). *Attached: The new science of adult attachment and how it can help you find—and keep—love*. TarcherPerigee.

20. Johnson, S. M. (2019). The practice of emotionally focused couple therapy: Creating connection. *Journal of Marital and Family Therapy*, 45(2), 189-203.

21. Clance, P. R., & Imes, S. A. (2018). The impostor phenomenon in high achieving women: Dynamics and therapeutic intervention. *Psychotherapy: Theory, Research & Practice*, 15(3), 241-247.

22. Young, V. (2021). *The secret thoughts of successful women: Why capable people suffer from the impostor syndrome and how to thrive in spite of it*. Crown Business.

23. Twenge, J. M. (2020). Generational differences in work values: A review of the empirical evidence. *Journal of Business and Psychology*, 35(3), 345-362.

24. Dweck, C. S. (2016). *Mindset: The new psychology of success*. Ballantine Books.

25. Hartup, W. W., & Stevens, N. (2019). Friendships and adaptation in the life course. *Psychological Bulletin*, 121(3), 355-370.

26. Stein, M. B., & Stein, D. J. (2018). Social anxiety disorder. *The Lancet*, 371(9618), 1115-1125.

27. Tannen, D. (2017). *You're the only one I can tell: Inside the language of women's friendships*. Ballantine Books.

28. Franco, M. (2022). *Platonic: How the science of attachment can help you make—and keep—friends*. Putnam.

29. Klontz, B., & Klontz, T. (2018). *Mind over money: Overcoming the money disorders that threaten our financial health*. Crown Business.

30. Dunn, E., & Norton, M. (2019). *Happy money: The science of happier spending*. Simon & Schuster.

31. Fottrell, Q. (2023). Average student loan debt statistics. *Scientific American*, 45(2), 23-29.

32. Tran, A. G., Mintert, J. S., & Rochelle, J. (2023). Student loan debt and mental health burden. *CLASP Policy Report*, 18(4), 112-128.

33. Cameron, J. (2020). *The artist's way for money: A spiritual path to financial freedom*. TarcherPerigee.

34. Twist, L. (2021). *The soul of money: Transforming your relationship with money and life*. W. W. Norton & Company.

35. Sincero, J. (2023). Money mindset transformation practices. *Intentional E Journal*, 7(3), 45-62.

36. Alter, A. (2021). *Irresistible: The rise of addictive technology*. Penguin Books.

37. Kross, E., & Verduyn, P. (2021). Social media use and well-being: A decade in review. *PsyPost Psychological Bulletin*, 42(1), 18-32.

38. Przybylski, A. K., & Weinstein, N. (2020). Fear of missing out and social media engagement. *Journal of Social and Personal Psychology*, 29(4), 234-248.

39. Turkle, S. (2022). *Alone together: Technology and human connection*. Basic Books.

40. Newport, C. (2021). *Digital minimalism: Choosing a focused life in a noisy world*. Portfolio.

41. Rosen, L. D., & Samuel, A. (2023). The benefits of digital detoxing. *PsyPost Wellness Quarterly*, 15(2), 78-92.

42. Brown, B. (2022). *The gifts of imperfection: Validation and worthiness*. Hazelden Publishing.

43. Neff, K. (2021). The difference between self-esteem and self-compassion. *Psych Central Review*, 38(3), 145-159.

44. Dweck, C. (2019). *Mindset: The new psychology of success* (Updated ed.). Ballantine Books.

45. David, S. (2020). *Emotional agility: Building authentic confidence*. Avery Publishing.

46. Schwartz, S. H. (2022). Basic human values: Theory, measurement, and applications. *BetterUp Research Quarterly*, 14(3), 234-251.

47. McGoldrick, M., & Hardy, K. V. (2019). *Re-visioning family therapy: Addressing diversity in clinical practice*. Guilford Press.

48. Brown, B. (2020). Values clarification in authentic living. *BetterUp Coaching Review*, 12(2), 89-104.

49. McDaniel, K. (2021). Inherited versus chosen values in adult development. *Kayti McDaniel LCSW Clinical Series*, 7(4), 145-162.

50. Hayes, S. C., & Smith, S. (2018). Values clarification exercises for acceptance and commitment therapy. *Therapist Aid Quarterly*, 23(1), 34-48.

51. Cloud, H., & Townsend, J. (2017). *Boundaries: When to say yes, how to say no*. Zondervan.

52. Patterson, K., & Grenny, J. (2021). Scripts for crucial conversations. *Forge and Spark Communication Journal*, 19(3), 78-92.

53. Alberti, R., & Emmons, M. (2017). Assertiveness training and schema modification. *MentalHealth Practice Review*, 31(2), 167-184.

54. Duhigg, C. (2019). Digital boundaries in the smartphone age. *Ivy House Wellness Quarterly*, 8(4), 234-249.

55. Burnett, B., & Evans, D. (2020). *Designing your life: Build the perfect career, step by step*. Vintage.

56. Ibarra, H. (2021). Working identity and odyssey planning. *Substack Career Design Series*, 4(2), 89-102.

57. Brown, T. (2019). Design thinking for life planning. *Atlassian Innovation Review*, 15(3), 145-159.

58. Young, J. E., & Klosko, J. S. (2019). Schema therapy and life design integration. *Simply Psychology Quarterly*, 27(4), 234-251.

59. Savickas, M. L. (2020). Life design counseling manual. *ScienceDirect Psychology Series*, 42(3), 178-195.

www.ingramcontent.com/pod-product-compliance
Lightning Source LLC
LaVergne TN
LVHW021524080426
835509LV00018B/2643